THE
URINARY INCONTINENCE
SOURCEBOOK

THE URINARY INCONTINENCE SOURCEBOOK

BY
DIANE KASCHAK NEWMAN,
R.N.C, M.S.N., C.R.N.P., F.A.A.N.

WITH
Mary K. Dzurinko

FOREWORD BY
Ananias C. Diokno, M.D.

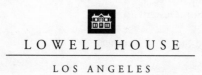

LOWELL HOUSE
LOS ANGELES

CONTEMPORARY BOOKS
CHICAGO

Library of Congress Cataloging-in-Publication Data

Newman, Diane Kaschak.
    The urinary incontinence sourcebook/by Diane Kaschak Newman
        p.   cm.
    ISBN 1-56565-648-2
    1. Urinary incontinence.   I. Dzurinko, Mary K.   II. Title.
    [DNLM: I. Urinary Incontinence.   WJ 146 N5519u 1997]
    RC921.I5N48   1997
    616.6'3—DC21
    for Library of Congress   97-6722
                                                              CIP

Requests for such permissions should be addressed to:

    Lowell House
    2020 Avenue of the Stars, Suite 300
    Los Angeles, CA 90067

Lowell House books can be purchased at special discounts when ordered
in bulk for premiums and special sales. Contact Department TC at the
address above.

Publisher: Jack Artenstein
Associate Publisher, Lowell House Adult: Bud Sperry
Director of Publishing Services: Rena Copperman
Managing Editor: Maria Magallanes
Text design: Robert S. Tinnon Design

Manufactured in the United States of America
10 9 8 7 6 5 4 3 2 1

To my family who made many sacrifices
so that I could have time to write:

My husband, Michael, who has supported my journey
through this field with his steadiness,
belief, understanding, and love.

My three remarkable girls—my angels—Carolyn Beth,
Michelle Amelia, and Emily Joellis, may they
grow a healthy, strong mind and body.

CONTENTS

ACKNOWLEDGMENTS

Special thanks to my colleagues who are experts in the field of incontinence and who shared their time and knowledge. I feel it is important that I single out their contributions and expertise because without their assistance and guidance I could not have finished this book.

Dr. Ananias Diokno, who wrote the foreword, is a personal friend and leading expert in the field of urology, particularly urinary incontinence. I had the privilege of working with him as a panel member on the 1992 AHCPR urinary incontinence clinical practice guideline where he was the co-chair of this expert panel. Since then he has included me in his international work with the Japan-U.S. Urology Group. I feel honored that he has chosen me to represent nursing and alternative treatment options in this international arena. His leadership and insight were invaluable to this endeavor. Dr. Diokno is Chief of Urology at Beaumont Hospital in Royal Oak, Michigan.

A very special acknowledgment to Nancy Reilly, R.N.C., M.S.N., A.N.P., nurse practitioner who has a continence practice in Toms River, New Jersey. She has been a steadfast friend throughout my career and through personal trials and tribulations. Her wisdom and knowledge in the urology nursing field is unsurpassed.

My gratitude to Kathleen McCormick, Ph.D., R.N., F.A.A.N., Agency for Health Care Policy & Research, who painstakingly reviewed this book for consistency and accuracy. As the co-chair of the 1992 AHCPR UI guideline panel of experts and nurse expert on incontinence in long-term care, Kathleen has been my mentor.

Deep appreciation to Joyce Wallace, R.N.C., M.S.N., C.R.N.P., adult nurse practitioner; Nicole Blackwood, R.N.C., M.S.N., C.R.N.P., geriatric nurse practitioner; Cathy Spencer, R.N.C., M.S.N., C.R.N.P., geriatric nurse practitioner; Karen Fritzinger, R.N.C., M.S., A.N.P., family nurse practitioner; and my staff and colleagues who reviewed, edited, and supplied me with their patient "stories" so that readers would understand what life is like living with the fear of urine loss.

I also acknowledge my nursing colleagues who are nationally recognized continence nurse experts in this field through their research, clinical, and government practice. They include: B.J. Czarapata, R.N., C.U.R.N., Urology Wellness Center, a nurse practitioner in private practice in Maryland; Sheila Fiers, R.N., B.S.N., C.E.T.N., an enterostomal therapist nurse specialist in Rochester, Minnesota; Mary Palmer, R.N.C., Ph.D., F.A.A.N., professor at the University of Maryland; Joyce Colling, Ph.D., R.N., F.A.A.N., professor, Portland, Oregon; and Dot Smith, R.N., M.S., C.E.T.N., C.O.N., F.A.A.N., Cheyenne Mountain Rehabilitation.

Special thanks to my physician colleagues and continence experts: Dr. Chris Steidle, Northeast Indiana Urology/ACCT Indiana, who gave me valuable information on the surgical side; Dr. Guy Bernstein, Bryn Mawr Urology, Bryn Mawr, Pennsylvania, who allowed me to borrow those special books on IC and bedwetting; and Dr. Andy Fantl, urogynecologist in Long Island who attested to my expertise.

Added gratitude to Kim Rowe of Rowe Marketing, New Jersey, for editing with intensity. Kim's review of management of UI was invaluable to providing the most accurate and current information.

I would like to acknowledge certain individuals in the manufacturing side who responded so quickly to my frantic calls for pictures, illustrations, and information: Al Mannino and Jim Carper, Rochester Medical; Phyllis Wilson, ConvaTec; Mary Pat O'Connor, Kimberly-Clark; Diane Gallagher, Jim Lutz, 3M; UroSurge; Elaine Austin, Humanicare; Jeannie Howard and David Hill, Coloplast; Benson Smith and Anthony Foote, C.R. Bard; Elizabeth Scarborough, Dan Habecker, and Lynn Brown, Mentor; Jackie Barrows, Uromed; Andre Contrefello, Mölylncke; Clara Kimbro, Health Services Research & Development; Linda Asta, A+ Medical Products, Inc.; Tom Hay and David Pollack, Bard U.K.; Sheryl Knapp, American Medical Systems; Randy Stern and Patti Gable, Standard Textile; Joy Boarini, Hollister; Jim Stupar, Incare; Melinda Early, Caring Products; Tom Abernethy, TransAqua; Brad Nelson, Sierra Laboratories; and Jan Kolmar, Empi.

During the writing of this book, my coauthor Mary Dzurinko was a true advocate for those suffering with UI and their caregivers. Through her research and editing she helped make this highly technical subject consumer friendly.

Last, but far from least, this book would not have been published without my editors Bud Sperry, who said yes to this project after many rejections because of the "sensitivity of the topic," and Maria Magallanes, for her calm and patience.

Finally, in the moral support department, besides my husband Michael Newman, special thanks to my brother and associate Joseph Dzurinko.

FOREWORD

Urinary incontinence is a worldwide condition that has no geographic boundaries. Millions of Americans are suffering from loss of bladder control. Once an ignored topic, the high prevalence of urinary incontinence (UI) in the United States was acknowledged after a 1982 landmark household survey which showed that 30 percent of men and women sixty years and older experience urinary incontinence.

During the last decade, tremendous advances have occurred in the management of urinary incontinence. These advances have occurred as a result of the contributions of support and knowledge from various government agencies who have been instrumental in promoting urinary incontinence. Many thanks to the National Institutes of Health (NIH), and specifically to the National Institute of Aging (NIA), for recognizing in the early 1980s the importance of urinary incontinence and providing significant research impetus toward the understanding, evaluation, and treatment of urinary incontinence. In response to the surge of knowledge regarding UI, the Agency for Health Care Policy and Research (AHCPR) convened a team of multidisciplinary specialists who wrote the first clinical practice guidelines for urinary incontinence in adults in 1992, which were subsequently updated in 1996.

Recognition should also be given to volunteer organizations and the corporate community for elevating public awareness of urinary incontinence. Two outstanding examples of nonprofit organizations, Help for Incontinent People (now the National Association for Continence) and the Simon Foundation, should receive special mention for their magnanimous efforts. The corporate community has also met the challenge by investing time and money to research and market diagnostic equipment, therapeutic devices, and pharmaceuticals, all essential management tools for clinicians and consumers alike.

As you will see, teamwork is an ongoing theme in this book. We have come this far today, not only because of funding from government agencies and the support of the community, but also due to the efforts of many scientists and clinicians who have devoted their careers to unraveling the many nuances of urinary incontinence. It is with great pleasure that I recognize the author, Diane K. Newman, for her numerous contributions to the field of urinary incontinence over a span of a decade. As a private nurse practitioner who has fully devoted herself to the field of incontinence care and treatment, Newman is uniquely qualified to write this book.

The Urinary Incontinence Sourcebook is extremely timely as consumers are now beginning to come out of the closet in search of solutions. With so many options available, caregivers are in need of access to information that is clear and concise. Newman explores the issues from A to Z and provides answers in her usual "say it like it is" style. By detailing anatomy and function of the lower urinary tract as well as the various symptoms and causes, this book leaves readers with an understanding of incontinence and informs them regarding the assessment of various types of UI. Newman then walks you through the many therapy options. The section on behavioral therapy is very well presented, and an encyclopedia of pads and pants, catheters, pessaries, toilets, commodes, and a list of product suppliers should prove helpful not only to consumers, but to caregivers as well. Although Newman's first choice in managing urinary incontinence is behavioral techniques, the author is thorough in her coverage of pharmacological and surgical treatment options.

It is my hope that this book will receive wide circulation. It is an excellent resource for consumers experiencing bladder control problems, relatives or significant others of incontinent patients, and students and practitioners of bladder dysfunction. The encyclopedic style of her book lends itself to be an excellent reference material in the home, office, clinic, and library.

ANANIAS C. DIOKNO, M.D.
CHIEF, DEPARTMENT OF UROLOGY
WILLIAM BEAUMONT HOSPITAL
ROYAL OAK, MICHIGAN

INTRODUCTION

In 1985 while in the process of completing my master's degree in nursing, I began looking for new challenges. I resigned from a nursing position I had held for over ten years and accepted an offer from a urologist friend to work with him on the development of a "continence center." As my previous nursing experience was in the area of kidney transplants, "bladder problems" were something familiar to me.

In the first month I was confronted by the limitations of the approaches and solutions to incontinence, the unwanted loss of urine. Incontinence has devastating effects on both men and women. Women clients returned for follow-up office visits after bladder suspension surgery, reporting that their incontinence was worse or had not improved. Men and women complained, "The medication the doctor gave me caused such a dry mouth that I can't talk," or "My constipation is worse now than before I started that drug." I quickly realized that the usual treatments for urinary incontinence were not the panacea that the medical profession thought they were. Unfortunately, I had no better answers. As a nurse and a mother I was used to "diapers" as the immediate solution to the problem of incontinence, but I had no real knowledge of what other incontinence treatments were available.

I set out to find some answers. During my research into the causes and treatments for urinary incontinence, I discovered behavioral therapy. Realizing the need for professional clinicians who could assess the problem, plan appropriate treatments, and introduce patients to incontinence management techniques, I set up a private practice in the Philadelphia, Pennsylvania area dedicated exclusively to the treatment and management of urinary incontinence. I published the results of my research and offered the specialized training programs I developed to other clinicians.

Over the past ten years, I have worked with persons with urinary incontinence and related problems such as interstitial cystitis, pelvic pain, constipation, and fecal incontinence. I have met women who save themselves from embarrassing situations at work by buying two skirts or two pairs of slacks in the same color and taking the extra set to work as a change of clothes if one set gets soiled. I have spoken with men and women who wet themselves while gardening, so they've stopped gardening. I've met others who wet themselves while genuflecting in church, so they don't go to church anymore. I have treated an eighty-five-year-old woman who keeps all of her windows open in summer and in winter because she's afraid that her apartment "smells." I have listened to the woman who doesn't have sex with her husband because of her fear that she'll have another "accident" during intercourse.

I have also seen the dramatic successes of my work. Women and men come back for a visit excited that bladder training has allowed them to make fewer trips to the bathroom. Patients who have followed my instructions on the use of bran in their diets get a new lease on life as their constipation problems improve. I have experienced deep gratification in aiding elderly caregivers to lessen their burden of caring for an incontinent spouse by switching to a product system designed to collect urine loss.

But I have also seen the stigmatization that "loss of bladder control" brings. Mothers and fathers hide it from their families for fear that their children will place them in a nursing home. Women, especially, who may first develop incontinence when pregnant, look at the problem as a nuisance, but something they have to live with. They wear sanitary pads every day "just in case," or to feel secure. Men, who experience incontinence as the result of a prostate condition, feel ashamed, and are reluctant to discuss the problem with family or their doctors. In the end, I've found that most people do not seek help and hide from their incontinence.

I wrote this book as a basic sourcebook for those who suffer with urinary incontinence and for people who love and care for them. As a medical professional, the mother of three daughters, and a member of a large family, most of whom are women, I am concerned about the lack of open, public discussion about urinary incontinence. The failure to actively seek and employ effective treatment and management programs by both individuals and the medical community annually adds astronomical costs to the U.S. medical economy. More importantly, urinary incontinence dramatically affects the quality of a person's life. I do not want women, in particular, to just live with it. I do not want women and men, no matter what their ages, to continue to suffer the "hidden taboo" in silence. I want them to demand answers from the medical community. This book is written for those of you who suffer with urinary incontinence and for those of you who provide care for incontinent individuals. It will help you take the first step to conquer and cure your condition by providing:

- a complete picture of what incontinence is and how it occurs,
- an explanation of your bladder and how it functions,
- information about dietary habits and exercises which affect incontinence, and
- details about therapies, medications, surgeries, and devices which cure and control urinary incontinence.

I want the reader to be aware that effective solutions to control and resolve urinary incontinence are available now!

And, I want to help the reader to realize the solution starts with you!

DIANE KASCHAK NEWMAN
NURSE PRACTITIONER

CHAPTER I

INCONTINENCE:
SERIOUS AND COSTLY

I n 1982, a column was published in "Dear Abby" that touched a nerve in thousands of people across the nation. Response from readers to that column was overwhelming. The subject was urinary incontinence (UI), the loss of bladder control, a condition currently affecting 17 million Americans. In frank terms, the column put the problem of incontinence squarely into the public eye and listed UI self-help groups' contacts and toll-free telephone numbers. That first column was just the beginning; over the last two decades, "Dear Abby" has highlighted urinary incontinence many times. In December 1992, the column included a letter from then Senator Bob Dole, the 1996 Republican presidential candidate. Senator Dole wrote about his prostate cancer and the urinary incontinence which sometimes results after prostate surgery. Again "Dear Abby" included information sources for readers. If there is a patron saint for persons suffering with incontinence, it may well be Abby!

Incontinence is an extremely expensive problem for consumers as well as the health care industry. In terms of dollars and cents, UI cost the United States health economy $28 billion ($3,941 per person) in 1995 and contributes to environmental pollution.

During the last ten years, the manufacture and sale of UI containment products, drugs, and devices have developed into a growth industry. Amazingly, adult diapers and absorbent products account for over 75 percent of the profits for companies producing such items; infant diapers and sanitary pads provide only 25 percent. In spite of the increasing problem, the National Institutes of Health spent only 7 percent of its 1995 research budget on diseases and conditions (Alzheimer's, urinary incontinence, diabetes, heart disease, Parkinson's, and so on) related to the aging process. Government experts predict the 1997–1998 budget will reduce funding for the National Institute of Aging by half. These decreases come at a time when greater numbers of baby boomers are beginning to join the senior population. Health care economists are very concerned by this trend. With their colleagues in the medical research community, they are exploring ways to cure, prevent, or reduce the number of people who have conditions such as incontinence. The American Federation for Aging Research and the Alliance for Aging Research estimate an annual savings of $8 billion if the onset of urinary incontinence could be delayed by just five years.

Adult diapers and pads, along with children's diapers, create serious trash disposal and health issues. The majority of the over 10 million used feminine hygiene pads, which are dumped daily into U.S. landfills, were used for containment of urine leakage. Of major concern to environmental and health experts is the fact that most of these materials are not recyclable; they create additional burdens for an already overburdened waste disposal system.

In the end, we all pay dearly for neglecting to control and treat incontinence with all available therapies.

SILENCE IS NOT GOLDEN

Rose has leaked urine, at least when she coughs or laughs, since her last baby was born in 1942. It wasn't an inconvenience; it was only a few drops each time, and using a small pad contained it. If her husband noticed that she had a problem, he never mentioned it. About ten years ago, when she broke her hip and had surgery to replace it, she began to lose urine on her way to the bathroom. It soaked through her pad to her pants. Rose is eighty-eight years old and afraid that her daughters will discover her secret. Her good friend and neighbor, Sue Walton, had the same kind of bladder problem, and Sue's sons sent her to a nursing home in a nearby town because of her urine odor. Rose doesn't want that to happen to her.

Until recently, UI was a secret problem, rarely disclosed by patients or openly discussed within families, and often undiagnosed and ignored by nurses and doctors. During the past decade, the treatment and care of UI have undergone a revolution. Media attention has brought urinary incontinence into the public spotlight. Newspaper, magazine, and TV coverage of the human and economic toll of urinary incontinence, as well as incontinent individuals and self-help groups such as the National Association for Continence, have contributed to public awareness. Incontinence information is also available in cyberspace—on the World Wide Web at the Wellness Web (http://www.wellweb.com/wellness) and from Internet discussion groups. Consumers should be aware that much of the information on the Web is questionable, but one reliable website is the Wellness Web.

The U.S. government has also played a part in heightening this new awareness. In 1992 the Department of Health and Human Services, Public Health Service, Agency for Health Care Policy and Research (AHCPR) issued its *Clinical Practice Guidelines on Urinary Incontinence in Adults* as part of a national effort to educate health professionals about the causes and available therapies for UI and to help them recognize patients who have it. In 1996 *Urinary Incontinence in Adults*, the first revised AHCPR guideline, was released. Although these guidelines may not, as yet, be widely utilized, they are the basis for building national programs to control and treat UI.

Chapter 2

HOW DOES YOUR BLADDER WORK?

Dorothy's bladder has always "ruled." Over the years she has learned the location of every rest room at the malls where she shops. Before driving from her house in Doylestown, Pennsylvania, to see her daughter in New Jersey, she always uses the bathroom. Dorothy says she has "weak" kidneys; her doctor once told her that her bladder is "the size of a kid's bladder." Not surprisingly, Dorothy, like most people, doesn't understand how her bladder works.

For many years *Readers Digest* published feature articles about human anatomy. Entitled "I am Joe's Brain," or "I am Joe's Heart," and so on, these features were written in lay terms and were very popular with readers. In fact, people who authoritatively quoted the information contained in them were said to have gotten their "medical degrees from the *Readers Digest!*"

Do you know the location of your kidneys? Do you know how your bladder works? Most of us are blissfully unaware of the part they play in our overall health until a kidney stone, a bladder infection, or urinary incontinence stops us. This lack of knowledge has special significance for incontinent individuals. It affects their attitudes about incontinence and may limit their participation in planning the treatment for their problem. So to help everyone start at the same point, here is the story of Mary's and Joe's urinary tracts.

THE KIDNEYS AND
THE URINARY TRACT STORY

Everyone has an upper and lower urinary tract system. (See Figures 2.1 and 2.2.) The upper system consists of two kidneys and two ureters. However, a person can live a perfectly normal life with just one of each. The lower urinary tract system contains the bladder, urethra, sphincters, and, in men, the prostate gland. The entire system is very complex, but you control it.

THE FILTERS: YOUR KIDNEYS

The kidneys and the ureters are in the upper urinary tract system. The kidneys are bean-shaped organs located on either side of the spinal cord behind your thirteenth rib. (See Figure 2.1.) People usually have two kidneys and each kidney has a ureter. The kidneys act as filters and eliminate wastes and water, called urine, from the blood. Elimination of wastes allows the body's basic functions—temperature, blood pressure, blood sugar, and so on—to remain in balance. The kidneys filter roughly 42 gallons of blood a day, but only about 1 percent of the blood's salts and water are passed out of the body in urine. Urine consists of approximately 95 percent water and 5 percent of the dissolved wastes (urea, creatinine, and uric acid) found in the blood. Nephrons, a set of very complex tubelike structures in the kidneys, delicately balance filtration, reabsorption, and secretion of the various elements of the body's fluids.

The kidneys constantly send urine to the bladder through two ureters, slender tubes approximately 9 inches long. Muscles in the ureters force the urine through the ureters with the aid of gravity. The urine is then collected in the bladder for later emptying.

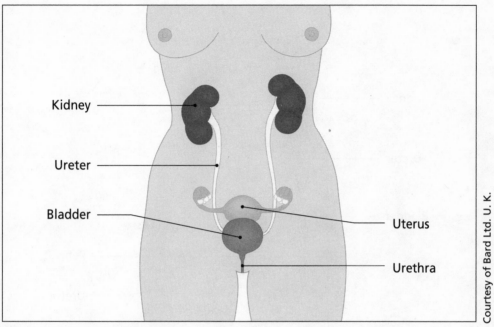

Kidney

Ureter

Bladder

Uterus

Urethra

Courtesy of Bard Ltd. U. K.

Figure 2.1 Female urinary system

THE STORAGE TANK: YOUR BLADDER

The lower urinary tract system contains the bladder and the urethra. This system is like a plumbing unit with a tank and a hose. The bladder is the tank and the urethra is the hose. Urine is temporarily stored in the bladder until it is passed through the urethra and out of the body. A rubber band–like structure, called a sphincter, keeps the urethra pinched so that urine does not escape. When a person decides to urinate, the sphincter relaxes and pressure in the bladder is increased; this assists in pushing the urine into the urethra and out of the body.

The bladder is a hollow muscle. It is like an elastic storage tank with a drainage tube (the urethra). Located in the pelvis behind the pelvic bone or,

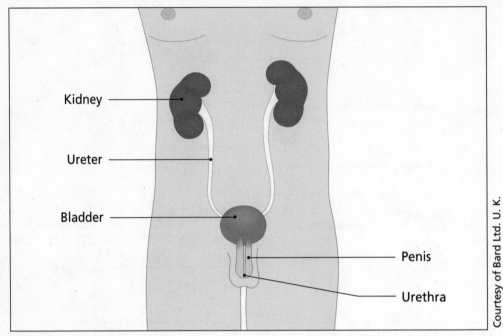

Courtesy of Bard Ltd. U. K.

Figure 2.2 Male urinary system

symphysis pubis, (see Figures 2.3 and 2.4), the bladder changes shape according to the amount of urine it contains. When empty, it resembles a deflated balloon. As the amount of urine in the bladder increases, it becomes somewhat pear-shaped and rises into the abdomen. The bladder is fully movable except at its base, or neck, where it becomes part of the urethra.

The bladder wall consists of three layers of muscle: the mucosa, submucosa, and detrusor. The mucosa is the innermost layer and the submucosa lies immediately next to it. The submucosa supplies the mucosa and its blood vessels with nutrients. The lymphatic in the mucosa helps remove waste products. The detrusor is a thick layer of smooth muscle which expands to store urine and contracts to expel it (see Figures 2.5 and 2.6). At the base of the detrusor muscle is the trigone, a triangular area located within the bladder wall. According to some scientists, the trigone may contain the sensory nerves of the bladder.

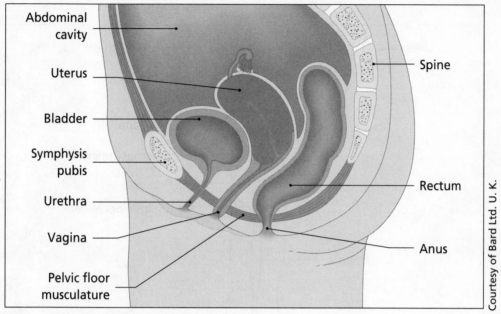

Figure 2.3 Female lower urinary tract (cross section)

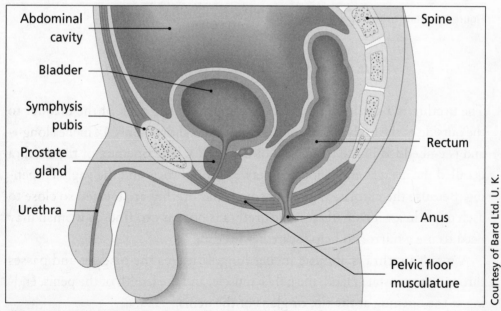

Figure 2.4 Male lower urinary tract (cross section)

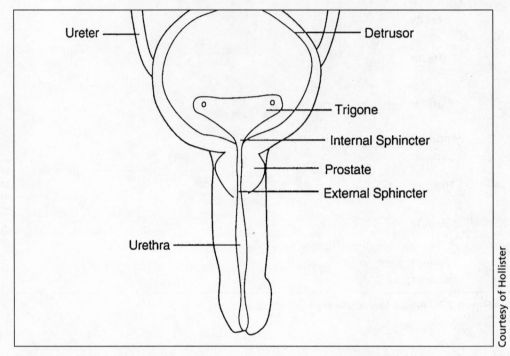

Ureter

Detrusor

Trigone

Internal Sphincter

Prostate

External Sphincter

Urethra

Courtesy of Hollister

Figure 2.5 Male urinary tract system

THE DRAINAGE TUBE: YOUR URETHRA

The urethra is a small, slender tube leading from the neck of the bladder to the outside of the body. In women the urethra is short—only 1½ inches long—and is embedded in the front wall of the vagina. The opening of the urethra is called the meatus and is located between the clitoris and the vaginal opening. Because the clitoris, vaginal opening, and urethra are located so close to each other in a very small area, the urethra is not easy to find. A woman may need to use a mirror to help locate her urethra.

A man's urethra is about 8 inches long. It leaves the bladder and passes through the prostate gland, the pelvic muscle, and the length of the penis, ending at the opening at the tip, or glans of the penis.

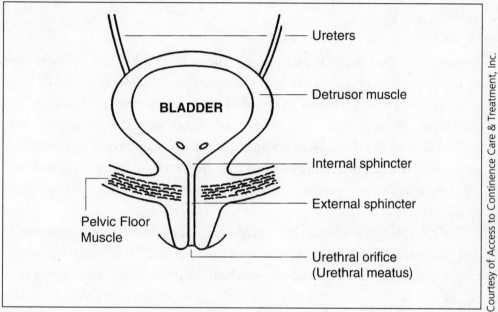

Ureters

Detrusor muscle

BLADDER

Internal sphincter

External sphincter

Pelvic Floor
Muscle

Urethral orifice
(Urethral meatus)

Figure 2.6 Female urinary tract system

THE MAINTENANCE ORGANS:
YOUR SPHINCTERS AND YOUR PELVIC FLOOR

Continence depends upon two factors—normal functioning of the bladder, urethra, sphincters, and pelvic floor muscle support.

THE BLADDER AND URETHRA

The bladder neck and the urethra are supported by a series of interconnected muscles and tissues called the pelvic floor muscles. These muscles, attached to the spine and pubic bone, keep the bladder, uterus, and rectum in place within the abdomen.

The Sphincters

Regulation of the storage and emptying of urine from the bladder is controlled by the internal and external urethral sphincters. A sphincter is a ringlike band of muscle fiber which closes off natural body openings such the anus and the urethra. Sphincters are supposed to stay tightly closed without your having to think about them. When you sit, stand, or walk, urine does not leak out of your bladder or urethra because your sphincters keep the urethra closed. The sphincters relax when messages are sent from your nerves and your brain to the pelvic floor muscles.

The internal sphincter is at the top of the urethra close to the bladder neck. The external sphincter lies below the internal sphincter. It is a smooth muscle mixed with the striated, or striped, muscle in the pelvic floor. You cannot consciously control smooth muscles. But the external sphincter's striated muscles allow for interruption of abdominal pressure. By interrupting this pressure, you can prevent urine leakage during activities—sneezing, coughing, blowing your nose, or laughing—that put pressure or stress on your bladder.

The internal and external sphincter muscles work closely together to control the various stages of bladder filling and emptying. The muscles around the bladder neck automatically expand and contract, holding urine in or letting urine out of the bladder. As the bladder fills, the nerves tell the muscles to keep the sphincter tightly closed and no urine is released. You are not aware of this message; it happens involuntarily with no conscious action on your part. However, at a certain point the internal pressure of the bladder becomes strong enough to stretch the bladder wall. A message is sent to the base of your brain through your nervous system. The brain then sends a message to the detrusor muscle in the bladder to automatically relax the internal sphincter. The external sphincter now consciously tightens and you feel a strong urge to urinate. When you have access to the toilet, you can relax the external sphincter muscle and urinate.

During the early stages of bladder filling, you are unaware of the slowly building volume of urine in your bladder, so you don't have to keep the external sphincter tightly closed. When enough fluid collects to relax the external sphincter, the urge to urinate occurs. The rectum also has a sphincter called the anal sphincter, which prevents bowel incontinence.

THE PELVIC FLOOR

In addition to sphincter muscles there are a series of interconnected muscle fibers and tissues that support the bladder neck and urethra called the pelvic floor muscles. These muscles are attached to your tailbone (coccyx) at the base of your spine and to the pubic bone at the front of your pelvis to keep the bladder, uterus, and rectum in place within the abdomen. This muscle is called the pubococcygeus muscle. The pelvic muscle consists of striated muscle fibers which are under voluntary control and can be exercised. Your pelvis supports your spinal column, which is attached to the rear of the pelvis. The bladder, urethra, rectum, and, in women, the uterus lie above and within the pelvic area. The pelvic floor surrounds, suspends, and anchors the pelvic organs, helping them remain in place. The pelvic floor is not a rigid platform, but strong, flexible muscles, often described as a "hammock." These muscles contract and expand during urination and bowel movements and distend during and contract after childbirth. The pelvic floor muscles can be used during intercourse for the sexual stimulation of a partner's penis. When infection or physical trauma damages the pelvic floor the tone, or firmness, and health of pelvic muscles and nerves are affected causing organs—the bladder neck (i.e., lower part of the bladder), urethra, or the uterus—to shift or sag. This puts unnatural pressure on pelvic floor muscles causing conditions such as incontinence or infection.

In addition to your sphincters and pelvic muscle, the prostate gland in men provides support for the pelvic floor. In women, the hormone estrogen helps keep the bladder, urethra, and muscles in the pelvic floor healthy and assists in maintaining good pelvic floor muscle tone. As a woman ages and goes through menopause her estrogen level drops, causing a loss of muscle support in the pelvic area.

IT'S ALL IN YOUR HEAD

Betty thinks there must be a connection between running water and her bladder. Every time she washes her hands, or the dishes, or the clothes, she wets her pants. Betty doesn't understand that there is not a nerve connection between running water and her bladder, but that it's "all in her mind." Betty's brain associates water with urine.

In simple terms, continence and incontinence are really controlled by your brain:

- The brain and central nervous system controls urinary bladder function.
- Continence or incontinence is controlled by messages exchanged between the brain and the body's muscle and nervous systems.
- Parts of the nervous system are located in the brain and along the spinal cord, as well as in nerves in the bladder and the sphincters.

The bladder, urethra, and pelvic muscles receive messages from the brain by two systems of nerves, the parasympathetic and the sympathetic. The parasympathetic system releases a chemical called acetylcholine: This stimulates receptors, called cholinergic receptors, in the body of the bladder, causing the bladder muscles (detrusor) to contract, allowing the bladder to empty. The sympathetic nervous system releases alpha-adrenergic and beta-adrenergic chemicals. The alpha-adrenergic substance affects receptors in the trigone of the bladder and in the internal sphincter. The beta-adrenergic substances stimulate receptors in the bladder body that result in smooth muscle relaxation of the bladder wall.

In the pelvic area, the pudendal nerve provides vital support for the pelvic muscles. The pudendal nerve has two branches—the forward branch goes to the urinary tract and the posterior branches to the intestinal tract, or the rectum. The nerve is like the trunk of a tree, sprouting branches of nerves out to the urinary tract and rectum.

As an infant, a person has little control over the urge to urinate. As the brain, muscles, and nerves mature, a "bladder control center" develops. Located in the front of the brain, the bladder control center controls the station located at the base of the brain which coordinates sphincter relaxation during urination. Urinary continence results when each system receives and correctly responds to the messages. Urinary incontinence results when there is a breakdown in communication between the bladder control center, the bladder, and the sphincters. This breakdown may be caused by either a mental or a physical impairment.

THE PATH TO NORMAL URINATION

The lower urinary tract is essentially a high-volume, low-pressure system. As long as the pressure within the urethra remains higher than the pressure within the cavity of the bladder, a person will be continent. Even when the bladder is full, it is elastic enough to accommodate additional fluid without causing pressure within the bladder. The bladder holds between 12 and 16 ounces of urine, about as much fluid as in a can of soda. Normally, an individual feels the urge to urinate when the bladder contains about 8 to 10 ounces of urine. The urge to urinate is an uncomfortable feeling or pressure that makes you want to empty your bladder. Usually, it indicates your bladder is full and needs to empty. However, in individuals who have frequent urination (urinating more than six or seven times per day) and incontinence, the bladder may not be full, but may be contracting and producing the urge unnecessarily.

Urination Patterns

There really are no "normal" urination patterns in the general population. Patterns which do exist range from every four to six hours to every eight to ten hours. Seniors over age sixty-five may urinate every three to four hours and at least once during the night. Bea's story is an example of what can happen within the bladder as you age.

> Bea had just turned seventy-two and was starting to feel old. She found herself going to the bathroom once an hour and getting up twice at night to urinate. Sometimes the "urge" came on so quickly that she was afraid she wouldn't get there if she didn't make a run for it. Many times she put a washcloth between her legs just in case she had an accident. When she told her family doctor about the problem, he just shook his head and cautioned her to be careful not to fall when she ran to the bathroom.

Bladder Changes with Aging

Bladder sensation changes with age. Seniors, instead of perceiving the bladder filling at half capacity as younger people do, may feel the need to urinate only when the bladder is almost full. To an active, mobile person, no matter what age, locating toilet facilities may be an inconvenience. To an immobile adult, a senior citizen, or an individual with an unstable bladder, "warning time" (the time between the realization of the need to urinate and the actual release of urine) is critical. Delay results in urinary accidents and, not infrequently, physical ones as well.

Another age-related bladder change is that bladder capacity is diminished. Overall the bladder muscle shrinks in size and cannot hold as much urine as it did at younger ages. Therefore, seniors feel the urge to urinate with lower bladder volumes.

> **Good Advice**
>
> **A**s an expert clinician in the field of incontinence, I have often heard my patients say, "Honey, you just don't understand, when I gotta go, I gotta go." Not true! Remember, you have a choice. Urination is voluntary and your bladder is under your control! So to go when you want to go, learn how!

Seniors produce their greatest volume of urine at night; two-thirds of their daily fluid intake is excreted at this time. This is because the kidneys make urine faster and more efficiently when people lie down and are at rest. The blood system pumps blood to the kidneys faster when the body is in a prone or supine position, and the kidneys are able to filter wastes more efficiently. Seniors may need to use the bathroom one or more times per night. These trips often produce falls and broken bones, especially in hips, legs, or arms. Seniors who do not completely empty their bladders make many trips to the bathroom each night.

Despite these age-related changes in her bladder, Bea shouldn't go to the bathroom every hour or every thirty minutes. No matter what your age, the bladder retains its flexibility. It can expand and hold urine through a concert or church service. The bladder retraining techniques discussed in Chapter 14 can help you maintain bladder control.

CHAPTER 3

THE BEST UNKEPT
HIDDEN SECRET

I f you suddenly became incontinent, wouldn't you recognize that you had a serious medical condition and seek help immediately? Or would you hesitate to visit your doctor because of feelings of confusion, shame, and fear? Or would you live with the problem and just try to handle urine leaks as best you could? We would like to think that every woman and man who has a problem with unwanted leakage of urine seeks help. Sad to say, that is not the case.

The first barrier to seeking help is the difficulty of admitting that you are incontinent. Since UI usually starts out as a slight problem (just a few drops), most people don't view it as a continence problem. When the condition gets worse, which it is apt to, you may be ashamed and lack the courage to tell family, friends, or even your doctor. Hesitation not only prolongs an incontinence problem, it brings unnecessary health care complications and costs.

WHAT IS URINARY INCONTINENCE?

Urinary incontinence is the cause of the smell that assaulted Sally as she entered the Red Hill North nursing facility. A registered nurse who worked temporary assignments, Sally knew that smell—urine. Obviously, the Red

Hill facility did not take enough care to ensure that bedridden residents were kept dry or that ambulatory residents were able to reach the bathrooms and use the toilet facilities.

Urinary incontinence caused the accident that Roberta couldn't believe happened to her. At age twenty-eight she had two children and loved to do aerobics and power walking. Her last child was a big baby, delivered after twenty-six hours of labor and three hours of pushing. In order to deliver the baby safely, the doctor had to "cut her." During her last exercise session, she wet herself while doing jumping jacks. Luckily she was wearing black running shorts so no one noticed. She has resorted to wearing feminine hygiene pads under her leotard.

Urinary incontinence is the cause of Abie's strained relationship with her daughter Sue. At age seventy-four, Abie doesn't appreciate being treated like a child. Sue is always badgering her about getting to the toilet in time, telling Abie that the chair she sat on is wet, or nagging about the bad odor that clings to Abie's clothes. Just wait until Sue gets old like me, Abie thought, she'll see what it's like.

Urinary incontinence is the accidental or unwanted loss or leakage of urine, or urinating when you don't want to do so. It is also commonly referred to as "loss of bladder control." Incontinence can vary from person to person, from day to day, occurring rarely or frequently. The amount of urine loss can be a few drops or as much as a cup. Most experts in the field describe incontinence in three degrees: light, moderate, or severe.

At some time in our stressful, active, and hectic lives, we all may experience an incident of incontinence. A visit to the doctor usually clears up the underlying problem and we quickly regain continence. When that incident develops into a pattern of leakage or flow serious enough to disrupt our lifestyles and daily routines and we don't get immediate medical assistance, it becomes a urinary incontinence condition.

UI is not a normal condition, nor is it a disease. Incontinence is a symptom of a bladder problem or the result of side effects of medications or an illness. A chronic medical problem, it can disable even a young person. It is feared by those who suffer with it, unrecognized by many medical professionals, and generally misunderstood by the public. Health professionals estimate that UI af-

Good Advice

Should you have a sudden and unexpected rush of urine, see your doctor immediately. It may be a sign of a serious medical problem.

fects more Americans than any other medical problem, condition, or disease. It is a major cause of institutionalization of the elderly, second only to dementia.

Many factors contribute to an incontinent symptom. Aging, pregnancy and childbirth, prostate cancer, loss of estrogen after menopause, physical and mental disabilities, medication, and surgery can cause loss of pelvic muscle tone and nerve damage. When the bladder loses its firm shape, shrinks, or drops from its correct position in the pelvic area, it relaxes, allowing urine to dribble or flow out in a stream. Usually a person is unaware that urine leakage is about to happen.

AN IGNORED RISK

A wide range of therapies and management techniques are available to help individuals like Roberta and Abie. However, although over 80 percent of treated cases have successful outcomes, most individuals do not seek treatment for their incontinence. In a survey of its members, the National Association for Continence found that men sought treatment within a year and a half after their incontinence appeared, probably because most men's incontinence occurred after prostate surgery.

Women, on the other hand, waited for three and a half years before seeking help. Studies show that women often view unwanted leakage of urine as part of being female; just another nuisance to deal with. Joy's story proves that point and suggests that a woman should check with her doctor any time she has an incident of incontinence:

Joy, a fifty-year-old postmenopausal career woman, was advised by her doctor to begin an exercise program to keep in shape and strengthen her bones. She enjoys a daily run, but has started to leak drops of urine during it. Her friend Selma said, "Don't worry, it's normal for a woman your age who exercises. That's what those thin panty-liner pads are for."

For women, high-impact exercise such as running and high-impact aerobics (especially jumping with legs apart) results in more episodes of incontinence than other sports. High-impact movements subject the pelvic floor to forces three to four times a woman's body weight, and pelvic floor ligaments cannot sustain these high forces for prolonged periods. They may become further damaged, especially if a woman already has weak pelvic muscles. The amount of urine loss depends on the mechanical pressure. This may explain why young women who have never been pregnant become incontinent during sports. Low-impact activities in which one foot is always on the floor allow women to exercise without urine loss. Panty-liners are not the answer; strengthening the pelvic floor is. See Chapter 14 and Appendix E.

Other studies indicate that some individuals wait from seven to nine years before they ask for medical help! Personal shame and fear, ignorance about incontinence treatments and their success rates, and family and societal pressures lie behind this hesitant attitude.

THE LAST TABOO

I recently had a very disturbing conversation with my friend Cathy. She was helping her mother wash a load of clothes and noticed that the clothes had a slight urine odor. Cathy asked if this might mean that her mother had a bladder problem. I asked her if she had discussed her concerns with her mother. Cathy explained that her mother is a very private person who has always been concerned about her personal health. Cathy felt that if her mother wanted to discuss a bladder control problem, she would bring it up herself and would be very upset if one of the family asked her about it. Cathy mentioned that her mother probably knew what was best for herself.

Cathy's views are not unusual. Most people don't want to interfere or intrude in a family member's most personal matters.

Until the 1990s, there was virtually no public discussion of urinary incontinence. Being incontinent is embarrassing, and incontinence is not a subject for polite conversation. More unfortunately, it was not even a subject at most patient-doctor interviews. Doctors had, and many still do have, an attitude of "Don't ask and don't tell." In the case of female patients, some doctors, inattentive to the special health needs of women, did not recognize urinary incontinence as a unique condition. As a result, they did not diagnose it. Older patients were reluctant to mention their condition to doctors and nurses because they believed that it was just the natural result of aging. Even some doctors and nurses viewed UI as an "old age" condition. Other patients, lacking knowledge about the functioning of their bodies and misunderstanding what incontinence is, believed there was no treatment for incontinence and there was no use bothering the doctors and nurses about it. Instead, they either ignored their problem on the theory that it would resolve itself, or they substituted incontinence products, such as diapers, for medical help. They "self-managed" their incontinence.

THE TABOO GOES PUBLIC

Today the subject of urinary incontinence is publicly and openly discussed on a national level. One of the crucial elements causing this change was the education of health professionals—doctors, nurses, physical therapists, and pharmacists. The urinary incontinence educational program went into high gear in 1992 when the Agency for Health Care Policy and Research (AHCPR) panel of experts issued an initial clinical practice guideline, Urinary Incontinence in Adults, along with a consumer guide. (Revised guidelines were issued in 1996.)

Today the public is subtly bombarded with TV and print ads for continence products. Hollywood stars (always women, you'll notice) from the forties and fifties hawk adult diapers during daytime soap operas, nightly news hours, and prime time sitcoms. Ads suggest that sanitary pads are useful not only for menstrual flow, but for other, meaning incontinence, "accidents." Campaigns highlighting the incidence of prostate cancer in men mention urinary incontinence as a possible result of prostate operations. Patients, including Michael Korda in his book *Man to Man: Surviving Prostate Cancer*, intimately describe their incontinent conditions.

Today the mention of incontinence to colleagues or friends brings quiet confidences that one's mother/husband/daughter has or had incontinence problems. Everyone seems to have had a personal encounter with urinary incontinence. Searching the Internet brings information about incontinence and incontinence management products to your desktop computer. Subscribing to wellness/health/cancer e-mail lists allows persons with incontinence to share successful and failed treatments and news of recent research. Medical and nursing practices specializing in urinary incontinence are springing up across the country. A multitude of self-help books and videos on incontinence are on sale in both general and health specialty bookstores. The taboo has gone public in the nineties!

But realistically, urinary incontinence is still the best-kept hidden secret of the nineties. Why else would so few people seek immediate help? Why else would so many people put up with the inconvenience of diapers and pads when there are effective therapies for UI treatment? The key to bringing the secret "out of the closet" lies in educating the incontinent person, the medical community, and the public about the causes, the burdens, and the treatment of urinary incontinence.

Chapter 4

THE BURDEN OF INCONTINENCE

No man is an island . . .

—John Donne

Urinary incontinence is both a community health problem and a personal crisis. You don't bear the burdens of urinary incontinence by yourself. The consequences to society at large (environment, health care costs, and so on) of UI are shared by your doctors and nurses and by your family and friends.

INCONTINENCE AND SOCIAL DYSFUNCTION

Since Bill had surgery nine months ago, he leaks urine (only drops) sometimes when he stands and always when he golfs. Bill is obsessed with going to the bathroom. All of a sudden the urge to urinate comes on, and Bill loses urine if he can't get to a john in a hurry. Before surgery, he golfed every day, but now he goes out only once or twice a week with friends who've also had prostate surgery. They tolerate his frequent need to relieve himself and his occasional stops because of a "large accident." Other guys just don't understand.

Persons like Bill isolate themselves from others through worry and humiliation. They go to great lengths to hide their problem. They can't, or believe they can't, tell others about it without receiving pity from those closest to them. They don't visit with friends because they can't sit still long enough to play one hand of bridge without jumping up to go to the toilet. They are uncomfortable at parties and dinners, fretting that an odor of urine surrounds their clothes and bodies. When they wear pads or diapers, they have the constant fear that urine will leak onto outer garments and furniture. Some wash underclothes and sheets by hand to hide urine stains from the people who do their laundry. Sleep deprivation is also common among incontinent individuals, who wake themselves up several times a night to make trips to the bathroom. Others worry that there will be no place to change their clothing should they have an accident. Some rarely attend church services; others give up movies and the theater. Even long-standing relationships are broken, sometimes never to be mended again. The consequences of an incontinence problem creep into every part of life.

TRAVEL

WHERE IS THE RESTROOM?

Several years ago Ida T. was referred to our urinary incontinence practice by a case manager social worker from the Philadelphia Corporation for Aging. Ida T. was a ninety-five-year-old widow whose only outside excursion was a weekly bus trip to Atlantic City to play the slots at the casino. For $10 she got a free bus ride and $10 in quarters, so it was a bargain, and she had been making the trip for over two years. However, during a visit with Ida, the social worker discovered that she had stopped going to Atlantic City. Her reasons were very vague. The social worker noticed that Ida T. had a bag of Depends® in her bathroom and asked her if she was experiencing any bladder problems. Ida T. said that yes, she was, but that it wasn't a new problem. Ida T. agreed to see an expert and came to our office. She didn't think of it as a problem. During our interview with her, we determined that Ida had been leaking urine. What she did see as a problem was the bus trip to Atlantic City. Once she arrived at the casino, she had to hurry to get a stool in front of a slot machine. However, after sitting on the bus for two hours, she really needed to empty her bladder. The ladies' room lines were so long that if she waited in them, she lost her chance at a slot stool. Several times she chose the stool over the bathroom and had a large bladder accident. She even leaked urine through her Depends® pads. She carried extra pads, but if she left her stool to change a pad, it would be hours before she found another one. Ida T. didn't feel that the trip was worth all the effort and possible embarrassment, so she stopped going.

Incontinent persons, like Ida T., view travel as an insurmountable obstacle. They make excuses and changes in their daily habits to ensure that traveling isn't part of their lives. When traveling on holiday, they try to ensure that their accommodations have appropriate access to a toilet. The concerns of men and woman differ when traveling. Men tend to be more concerned about urinary accidents on the journey or in bed, while women are most concerned about the availability of bathrooms. But most individuals with urinary incontinence pack special items when traveling—bedpads, linens, plastic bags, and rubber pants. One woman related that she used to pack one suitcase of clothes and one suitcase of pads for each business trip.

Vacations and excursions are curtailed, and even short trips away from home are avoided. Grocery shopping is an ordeal because of the absence of convenient rest rooms and worry about getting caught in a long line at the checkout counter. Incontinent individuals go to great lengths to make certain that they know where all the bathrooms are located. Travel brings the possibility that there won't be a rest room available when they need one. Mistakenly believing that if you don't drink, you won't wet, they don't drink any liquids for several hours before they do travel. They wear loose clothing and absorbent pads in case they have an accident.

The Lack of Public Toilets

Unlike Europe, the United States has very few public toilets in towns and cities. In a major European city like Glasgow, Scotland, clean and well stocked rest rooms are be found on major streets throughout the city. In the United States, city rest rooms are typically located in parks and recreation areas. Many of these are dangerous, dirty, and in disrepair. Highway sites are better, although rest stops are usually miles apart. Gas station rest rooms are kept locked to stop crime and vagrancy, and it's difficult to find the key or locate the person who has custody of it. In public theaters, stores, or crowded venues, facilities are no more convenient. And, as every female knows, there are never enough stalls in these places to accommodate the number of women.

20/20, the ABC television newsmagazine, had a feature in the spring of 1996 highlighting the inadequate number of stalls in women's rest rooms. Correspondent Lynn Sherr interviewed women at the symphony, in the U.S. Congress, on the street—they all said the same thing. They find themselves at these venues standing in line with scores of other women, and often uncomfortable, patiently waiting to use a rest room with five available stalls. The fact that women must remove some of their clothing and actually sit down and get up increases the time they spend using the toilet. Men, on the other hand, literally "zip" in and out of the rest room, yet men's rest rooms are usually the same size as women's.

These conditions change slowly. When Oriole Park at Camden Yards was built in the early 1990s as the home for the Baltimore Orioles baseball team, one of the stated architectural goals was to build sufficient rest room facilities. Even when an Orioles game is completely sold out, it's rare to wait in line at the door to a ladies' room. In late July 1996, New York City began reopening rest room facilities and building new public toilets. Over a thousand public rest stops are planned for locations throughout the city. In an urban environment, it will be a challenge to keep these facilities clean and safe, especially for women and children.

SEX

Intimacy is a personal and delicate act. The self-image of both sexes is intertwined with sexual performance. In the face of urinary incontinence, sexual activity is often restricted or completely avoided. Difficulty getting an erection, leakage of urine during orgasm, physical pain, bed-wetting, urinary tract infections, and loss of bladder control are personally embarrassing and humiliating. No one likes to take direct hits like these to the ego. Individuals who don't face their incontinence squarely usually can't communicate their fears and concerns to sex partners. Some couples begin to sleep separately without ever discussing the reason. If the partner's sense of smell is keen, all affectionate contact may cease, adding another negative consequence to an already distressing situation. Believing that by avoiding sexual intimacy their secret can be kept hidden, individuals cut themselves off from the best support they have to help cope with UI—a spouse or significant other.

It is truly unfortunate that so many feel they must face the burden of incontinence alone. So much care and help is available, especially if a person is supported by medical professionals and family and is encouraged to investigate incontinence therapies.

CARING FOR SOMEONE WITH INCONTINENCE

Paul has been taking care of Sophie in their apartment for the last two years. Sophie is a "total care" wife. She had a massive stroke two years ago, is confined to a hospital bed, and does not speak. When Paul tries to turn Sophie from her back to her side, she grabs his arm and scratches it. Sophie is totally incontinent and her incontinence is managed with a bladder catheter that collects the urine. Recently it began to fall out every two days, and now she wears diapers. Paul sleeps next to Sophie in a cot and changes his wife's diapers every two to three hours during the night so that her skin doesn't break open and ulcerate. Paul always looks tired, but if he's asked if the strain of caring for Sophie is too much for him, he always replies, "Sophie and I have been married for fifty years, and we've always said we'd take care of each other."

In all likelihood, every family has a member who has suffered from urinary incontinence, and that person is usually a woman. The 15 to 17 million Americans suffering from urinary incontinence are not just nursing home residents, although over 50 percent of nursing home residents are incontinent. At least 30 percent of the general adult population from every walk of life and with all kinds of physical and mental conditions experience incontinence. This necessitates a UI care system which can handle the needs of people of every social and economic status.

Adults associate wet underwear with childhood and children. If they become incontinent, they view it as the beginning of the loss of control over their lives. The possibility of being dependent on others for physical care or the decline of a productive life are difficult situations to face. If such worries become a dominant force in an incontinent person's life, he or she may forego prompt and proper care, causing further deterioration in physical and even mental health.

Then, too, all Americans are obsessed with personal hygiene. America undoubtedly has more brands of deodorant, mouthwash, and toothpaste than any other country in the world. This hygienic fixation contributes to an incontinent person's fear that the smell of urine will cling to him or her and makes maintaining dryness and cleanliness of paramount concern. Some might choose to manage incontinence by themselves, for instance, by using absorbent products, without investigating less expensive and more effective therapies. In many cases, this self-management prolongs the condition and creates more complicated problems.

Urinary incontinence is a burden for persons who experience it, but it also has a dramatic impact on the lives of families, friends, and caregivers. Many incontinent persons become depressed and, in time, develop severe psychological and physiological problems. Dealing with an incontinent, depressed parent or mate puts a strain on family relationships. Sufferers with physical limitations—walking difficulties, for example, or mental impairment—need special care. The family has a difficult time dealing with a stubborn, uncooperative individual who may have a negative attitude toward a UI problem. Additionally, availability and kind of care, along with economic concerns, play a large role in a family's ability to cope with an incontinent relative. These problems place constraints on the time and type of care and attention a family can expend.

As the aging population increases and home care becomes the norm, family members, especially women, who are the primary caregivers, need to have knowledge of incontinence treatments and how to get help. If you suspect that your mother or father is suffering with an incontinence, urinary urgency, or frequency problem, try different approaches to break her or his wall of silence. The current older generation was raised in a much more restrictive, puritanical time, and discussion of bodily functions was uncommon. In broaching the subject, acknowledge that it may be embarrassing and emphasize that you are not passing judgement but that you want to help find permanent solutions for the problem. One way to reduce your parent's or relative's embarrassment is to say, "You are one of 17 million Americans who have a problem with incontinence," or " In the over-sixty age group, four out of ten women and two out of ten men are troubled by loss of bladder control," or "I've learned of several therapies that could completely control or cure your incontinence." Caregiving is further discussed in Chapter 20.

CHAPTER 5

MYTHS

J ust like the tales of alligators in the city sewer system, there are lots of "urban myths" about urinary incontinence. An urban myth is a story with a moral, told by a friend who heard it from a friend's friend who swears it happened to his mother's cousin. Misconceptions about urinary incontinence fall into this myth category.

MYTH 1: "I'M JUST GETTING OLD"

Bodies change with age. We may gain weight, our skin may start to sag. One day we wake up to find we need a wider shoe size. Our hair may turn silver, then white, then may fall out completely. But incontinence is not an ordinary and inevitable part of this aging process.

However, there are physical and medical factors which affect a person's bladder sensations and awareness:

- Loss of the hormone estrogen by postmenopausal women may cause thinning of the tissues surrounding and supporting the pelvic area, resulting in incontinence.
- Enlargement of the prostate gland may inhibit the complete emptying of the bladder, causing a man's urine to leak or dribble out.

- Decreased bladder capacity may cause urinary urgency, leading to frequent toileting and incontinence in older adults.
- Susceptibility to infections increases with age and predisposes some seniors to symptoms of incontinence.
- Arthritis and diabetes, common ailments contracted in later life, may result in urinary incontinence.
- Alzheimer's and Parkinson's diseases, dementia, and senility may impair a person's mental ability. Communication lines between the brain and the bladder get crossed, and continence messages are not received by the pelvic floor's nervous system.
- Chronic medical conditions requiring multiple medications may further predispose seniors to urinary problems. The common use of multiple medications by the senior population is a most troublesome medical issue. When medications are not carefully prescribed and tracked, not only urinary incontinence, but mental confusion and serious health complications can be the result.
- Vision and mobility change as a person ages and may impair an individual's ability to get to a toilet in time. Many seniors cannot even use toilet facilities. (In one patient-related incident, a man wet his pants while attempting to figure out the 4-digit combination lock of a public rest room. The hallway was dark, and the man had decreased vision and dexterity.)

MYTH 2: "NOTHING CAN BE DONE ABOUT IT ANYWAY"

It ain't necessarily so! In most cases, incontinence can be treated successfully, with cure rates of up to 85 percent. Most people are unaware that help is available. Among the current ways to manage urinary incontinence are:

- behavior interventions
- diet modification
- bladder retraining
- Kegel or pelvic muscle exercises
- biofeedback therapy
- lifestyle modification
- medications
- surgery
- new technology to help with management

With careful treatment and attention, incontinence resulting as a complication of a disease such as diabetes may be completely reversible.

Hand in hand with this myth is the denial by some that they are, indeed, incontinent. Many see their condition as a short-term problem, certainly an inconvenience, but a situation that will probably resolve itself. For many people it is very difficult to deal with the reality of UI. When shame, fear, and outside pressures force incontinent persons into a defensive posture, they end up hurting themselves and their health.

MYTH 3: "I WON'T NEED SURGERY, WILL I?"

All of us are reluctant surgical candidates. Concerns that we won't wake up after an operation or that while under anesthesia, the doctors will do something that will leave us physically or mentally impaired, with the wrong organ removed, or dead, are high on the list of the fears of surgery. Seniors are very worried that if they discuss their incontinence with a doctor, surgery will immediately be suggested as the cure. Surgery for older adults is probably the last option for incontinence and is usually reserved for individuals for whom all other treatments have failed. However, in cases such as an enlarged prostate, surgery may be the best option.

MYTH 4: "I TRUST MY DOCTOR TO TELL ME WHAT TO DO"

The incontinent consumer has to depend on more than what a doctor or nurse says or does. UI is not a life-threatening condition, and it may not be seen as a serious problem by some doctors and nurses. Your doctor or nurse may not be aware of the available treatment options. On the other hand, medical professionals know that patients don't always supply all the information necessary to make a complete diagnosis. To get a complete history, clinicians use examinations, tests, observations, and interviews as tools.

An incontinence treatment plan involves physicians and nurses who investigate a patient's symptoms and map out a plan to control, improve, or cure incontinence. Nurses and therapists help the patient implement a care plan, adapt it to the patient's needs, and evaluate its success. Pharmacists review the patient's's drug regimen in order to determine the effectiveness of prescribed drugs and monitor the patient for adverse drug reactions. When institutionalization or home care is indicated, social workers advise the patient and other family members about home or facility care and the economic implications of care and treatment. A multidisciplinary approach to the treatment of urinary incontinence produces the best outcome for both patients and their families.

MYTH 5: "I'M SO CONFUSED"

Society's view of incontinent persons is that they are senior citizens who've lost control of their minds and bodies, the homeless who should all be in mental institutions anyway, and persons who are mentally ill. However, people of sound mind who belong to none of these groups also suffer from incontinence. Unfortunately, these individuals may not discuss their symptoms with a physician or seek treatment. They either accommodate their lifestyles to their incontinence or find other methods of managing it. Because of this, they are not in the count of the incontinent population, and it impossible to determine the real numbers of everyone who suffers with incontinence.

MYTYH 6: "ALL I NEED
ARE SOME DIAPERS"

June Allison was a popular actress and is an attractive salesperson for Depends®, the absorbent pads. However, she isn't the spokesperson for urinary incontinence—in the ads she doesn't explain what UI is, its causes, or any other treatments. Consumers should be clearly aware that the use of Depends® and diapers, pads, and absorbent underwear is not a cure for incontinence. Because it is so easy, many individuals first turn to the use of absorbent products conveniently found in drugstores, supermarkets, and discount stores without having their conditions properly diagnosed and treated. In the early stages of an incontinence problem or if treatment for incontinence is only partially effective, absorbent products are a valuable part of a treatment regimen. But the cornerstones of incontinence treatment are identifying the factors causing the condition and attempting to decrease the amount of urine that is involuntarily lost.

Chapter 6

CAUSES AND TYPES OF INCONTINENCE

Documented risk factors associated with incontinence are wide ranging . . .

—AHCPR Urinary Incontinence Guidelines

The AHCPR's (Agency for Health Care Policy and Research) 1996 incontinence panel of experts who updated urinary incontinence clinical guidelines define urinary incontinence as "involuntary loss of urine that is sufficient to be a problem." Urinary incontinence doesn't appear without an underlying cause. A person's incontinence may be directly connected to defined internal and external predispositions. These predispositions, or risk factors, affect the anatomy and physiology of the lower urinary tract. Changes or damages to pelvic floor muscles and nerves, the bladder, or the urethra can result in urinary incontinence.

PERSONS AT RISK

RISK FACTORS

The AHCPR expert panel documents the risk factors associated with incontinence as:

Restricted Mobility Commonly Associated with Chronic Diseases

Includes confinement to a bed or a wheelchair due to a disease such as arthritis or Alzheimer's disease, hip fractures which do not heal properly, or other surgical complications. Angie is an example:

Angie is eighty years old and was quite active until she broke her hip. She was always able to control her bladder, but since her surgery she's had two accidents because she can't get to the bathroom quickly enough. Getting up from the couch is difficult, and she now walks very slowly. In the hospital and rehab center Angie didn't realize she might have a bladder problem because she had a catheter in her bladder.

Change in Mental Status and Delirium

Includes dementia, mental illness, confusion, and depression. Ernie is an example:

Ernie has been experiencing memory loss for several years and his doctor told his family that Ernie may have Alzheimer's disease. Ernie is a widower and lives with his daughter, Pat. He has periodic episodes of urine and bowel incontinence and is very embarrassed when this happens. He says that it isn't his fault. The doctor told Pat that the incontinence may indicate that Ernie's Alzheimer's disease is progressing, and as his memory loss worsens, he probably won't remember where the bathroom is located and won't recognize the urge to urinate.

Medications, Including Diuretics

Includes use of multiple medications, sedatives, narcotics, and other drugs which diminish bladder sensation. As discussed in Chapter 2, the lower urinary tract, bladder, and urethra are controlled by your nerves and the bladder control center in the brain. So anything that alters, slows, or dulls the nerves or brain will affect your bladder. For example, if you have pain and take a pain medication, you will alter or delay the urge sensation or message sent by your brain telling you to empty your bladder. Judy is an example:

At age seventy-three, Judy has a difficult time sleeping. Usually she can't fall asleep till 2 A.M. and she's awake by 5 A.M. so her doctor gave her the sleeping pill Restoril. Judy is very concerned because although she now sleeps through the night, she has started wetting her bed. What Judy doesn't understand is that at age seventy-three her kidneys are producing the majority of her urine while she is resting. Therefore, more urine is dumped into her bladder during the night, but she doesn't know she has to urinate because the sleeping pill has dulled the message from her brain.

Smoking

Although it is documented that smokers have a greater likelihood of becoming incontinent than do nonsmokers, the relationship between smoking and incontinence is not well understood. It is thought that chronic smoker's cough may cause stress incontinence.

BOWEL IMPACTION

Stool impaction can cause urinary and fecal incontinence. Stool that has built up in your rectum over days and weeks hardens and puts increased pressure on your bladder, causing incontinence.

OBESITY

Being overweight can contribute to incontinence. Even a few pounds can make a difference. A 5 to 10 percent weight loss can significantly reduce the intra-abdominal pressure putting added stress or pressure on your bladder, causing leakage of small amounts of urine.

LOW FLUID INTAKE

Contrary to popular belief, maintaining adequate fluid intake is important, especially for older adults who already have a decrease in total body water and are at risk for dehydration. In certain cases, drinking the eight 8-ounce glasses of fluid per day may eliminate incontinence.

ENVIRONMENTAL BARRIERS

Persons who have mobility or balance problems may be unable to suppress an urge to urinate until a caregiver arrives to toilet them. If they are independent, they may be unable to walk or propel their wheelchairs to the toilet in a timely fashion. These individuals can benefit from convenient bathroom facilities and bedside commodes, sufficient lighting, and special bathroom fixtures such as railings, low toilets, and so on.

HIGH-IMPACT PHYSICAL ACTIVITIES

It is thought that at least 50 percent of women who exercise regularly experience some degree of stress incontinence. Usually, a woman will wear a tampon or panty liner, change her sport, or stop exercising altogether to cope with the incontinence. Certain physical activities cause increased pressure in the abdomen, thus increasing downward pressure on the bladder. If the urethra muscles are not tight, small amounts of urine leak out. Sports associated with increased pressure on the bladder include gymnastics (trampoline, floor exercises), combat sports (karate, judo), team games (basketball, tennis, volleyball, handball), horseback riding, bodybuilding with heavy weights, and track and field (jumping and running). Activities with little risk include swimming, bicycling, walking, rowing, low-impact aerobics, and others in which at least one foot touches the ground at all times. Incontinence related to sports is not age discriminate. A patient of mine recently told me that she has a seventeen-year-old sister who is an avid sports enthusiast, playing softball, hockey, and soccer. She has stress incontinence and wears pads all the time during practice and games.

Good Advice

If you fit into any of these risk groups and you suddenly have an incontinence incident or have suffered with incontinence for any period of time, consult your doctor immediately.

MEDICAL PROBLEMS—DIABETES, STROKE, ARTHRITIS

Illnesses such as diabetes actually interrupt the messages on the nerve pathways to the bladder, causing the bladder not to empty completely (urinary retention). Other illnesses (stroke, arthritis) may impair the ability of a person to get to the bathroom in time.

Loss of the Hormone Estrogen

There are hormone receptors in the bladder, urethra, and pelvic muscles. Once a woman goes through menopause, hormone levels of estrogen are reduced, causing atrophy (wasting) of tissues in the pelvic area. Symptoms of urgency, frequency, dysuria (difficulty in urination), and urinary incontinence may occur.

Pelvic Muscle Weakness, Pregnancy, Vaginal Delivery, and Episiotomy

Changes in the urinary system are common during pregnancy and may influence urinary control in some women. It is not uncommon for women who have previously had normal control to start having accidents while they are pregnant. Half of all women pregnant for the first time experience bladder control problems, especially during the last trimester. Bladder control problems may become more severe with each additional pregnancy. The strain of labor, vaginal delivery, and episiotomy (a procedure which involves cutting into the pelvic muscles) weakens pelvic floor structures. (See Figure 6.1.) Incontinence may persist after childbirth.

THE AHCPR GUIDELINES IN ACTION

The AHCPR guidelines clearly state that aggressive identification of candidates at risk for incontinence and implementation of recommended treatments resolve most incontinence conditions. According to the AHCPR expert panel, effective management of UI focuses on proper medical assessment of the patient and the incontinence condition, identification of the risk factors and causes of the in-

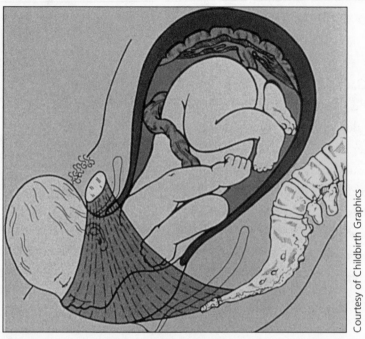

Courtesy of Childbirth Graphics

FIGURE 6.1 Pelvic floor muscles released at birth

continence, treatment of conditions which can be reversed, open discussion of all UI treatment options, development and implementation of a UI management program which fits a patient's desires and goals, and patient education. The AHCPR urges doctors and other health care providers to closely evaluate patients for incontinence problems and to monitor patients' bladder functions.

Types of Incontinence

The AHCPR expert panel identifies two basic types of incontinence: acute incontinence and chronic incontinence.

Acute incontinence is a temporary or reversible condition, related to an illness or a specific medical problem.

TRANSIENT CAUSES OF ACUTE INCONTINENCE

Marta got on the Gatwick Airport train at London's Victoria Station. A sixty-eight-year-old retiree, she was on her way home after a two-week tour of England and Wales. As she approached the British Air counter, everything let go in a rush. Her underpants were soiled and wet. She quickly found an airport rest room. Luckily, she still had her luggage with her and could change clothes. The flight was uncomfortable. Afraid that she'd have another accident, she made frequent trips to the lavatory to empty her bladder. Upon arrival in New York, Marta immediately went to her doctor, where tests confirmed she'd had a small stroke.

Good Advice

During your first visit to a continence professional, ask if he or she is familiar with and uses the AHCPR guidelines.

Marta developed incontinence seemingly out of the blue. But the condition was really a symptom of her stroke. Just as she could not anticipate the stroke, she couldn't anticipate the incontinence. Once her medical problem was resolved, her incontinence immediately improved and eventually disappeared.

ILLNESSES

Temporary incontinence sometimes appears during an illness. Faulty communication between the brain and the body's nervous system interrupts or confuses messages sent from the bladder control center to the bladder and sphincters. Perception of the need to urinate or the sensation of a full bladder diminishes or completely disappears. During an illness, dehydration may mask the need to urinate. Dehydration concentrates a person's urine inside the bladder, irritating the bladder wall and urethra and resulting in urinary frequency or incontinence. People who are ill are primarily concerned with their treatment and recovery. Bladder needs are not clearly or quickly recognized. Response to bladder sensations may be slow or ignored until the urge to urinate suddenly appears. In many cases, an incontinence incident is the first indication to an ill person that a bladder problem exists. When medical problems are resolved, incontinence is resolved, too.

As we've mentioned, advertisers would have us believe that diapers are the perfect answer for temporary incontinence. They are not a treatment, but only a stop-gap measure. In fact, they may deter or delay recovery because patients rely on them instead of actively working with their physicians, nurses, and families to resolve incontinence.

Men with prostate problems may retain urine in their bladders. An enlarged prostate causes narrowing and compression of the urethra. Blockage or an obstruction in the urethra can lead to urine leakage or temporary incontinence. Treatment depends upon the cause of the obstruction and the severity of the medical condition.

Physical disabilities—difficulty walking, inability to use legs, arms, or the upper/lower body, impaired hearing or eyesight—are obstacles to using the toilet. Recovery from surgery, serious illness, and bed rest also limit physical mobility and present additional challenges. Falling down is a great fear for older adults. Falling often occurs during the night when you may frequently attempt to get to the bathroom. It's frustrating to face what appears to be an insurmountable obstacle every time you have to use the toilet. If toilet facilities are not easily reached and accessible, if a portable bedside commode or urinal is not at hand, if no one is near to provide assistance in getting up and walking to a bathroom, sitting on a toilet, or using a bedpan, individuals grow frustrated in their attempts to do the best they can. They tend to "throw in the towel." These frustrations can lead to incontinence during some stage of their incapacity.

YOUR BOWELS' IMPACT ON
YOUR PROBLEM

Bowel problems may be a cause of temporary incontinence. Constipation, or fecal impaction, occurs when a large amount of fecal matter or stool
is lodged in the intestines and rectum. Hard stools
put pressure on the bladder, changing its position

Good Advice

Be careful—straining
causes damage to pelvic
floor muscles and nerves.

within the pelvic area and causing either incontinence or urine retention. In
order to resolve constipation, people strain or push to relieve their bowels.
If you are frequently constipated, review your diet for its fiber content and
amount of fluid intake and visit your doctor for a checkup. Once a normal
bowel movement takes place, a person is able to urinate and incontinence is
resolved. (We'll learn more about fecal incontinence later.)

BLADDER INFECTIONS AND INCONTINENCE

"I can't make it, it comes out too quick," complains eighty-two-year-old
Nellie P. Nellie was referred to the continence nurse specialist because she
had lost her bladder control after a recent hospital stay for a perforated stomach ulcer. Nellie told the specialist that she has a history of cystitis. Nellie
had a catheter in her bladder while in the hospital and it was removed before
she was discharged. Since she's been home Nellie feels that her urine "just
gushes out." When the nurse tested Nellie's urine she found that Nellie had a
bladder infection. Nellie was given antibiotics and her incontinence problem
stopped once the infection cleared.

A urinary tract infection (UTI), often called cystitis, is an indication of bacteria in the urine.

- UTI may be connected to a kidney infection.
- UTI may result from lax personal hygiene. Women should carefully clean themselves after each bowel movement, wiping front to back, so that bacteria from the rectum isn't transferred to the vaginal area.
- UTI may occur when using a diaphragm. A diaphragm is flexible, but its rigid ring can cause irritation. It should be throughly cleaned after use to remove any bacteria.
- UTI bacteria can be spread during sexual activity. An infection may be passed between sex partners and sexual activities may bruise the urethra or cause swelling and inflammation in the vaginal area.
- UTI is a greater risk for women than men because the female urethra is shorter making it easier for germs to go the smaller distance from the anus to the urethra.
- UTI is more common in older woman because of changes in the urinary tract which come with age and a less efficient immune system.

UTI irritates the bladder lining, causing you to feel the need to urinate more often even if there is only a small amount in your bladder. The infection usually causes urgency, urinary incontinence, and occasional pain or burning when urinating. A bladder dysfunction, such as an unstable detrusor (the detrusor is the bladder wall muscle and involuntary contractions or rising pressure in the bladder can cause instability) aggravates UTI. In younger and middle-aged adults doctors usually spot UTI immediately because the patient complains of burning sensations, frequent urination, fever, and lower back pain. Urinary incontinence is often a senior's only symptom of an infection. To determine the presence of a urinary tract infection, a urinalysis is done. If an infection is found it is treated with antibiotics, and incontinence and other bladder symptoms will resolve. If you are a person who has frequent UTI, acidifying your urine with vitamin C (ascorbic acid) may prevent recurrent infections. Women also report that cranberry juice helps. However, if you have irritative symptoms such as urgency, frequent urination, and burning when you pass your urine, cranberry juice might make these symptoms worse. Also, cranberry juice is high in calories.

Atrophic Vaginitis

Joellis stopped menstruating four months ago and since then has noticed problems with urinary urgency. She feels like she always has to go to the bathroom. Sex with her husband is uncomfortable because her vagina feels so dry. When she visited her nurse practitioner for her yearly Pap smear, the nurse mentioned that Joellis's vaginal tissue is thinner and she probably had atrophic vaginitis. The nurse practitioner recommended estrogen-based cream to keep the vaginal tissues moist and to keep the muscles toned. The estrogen would help the tissue of her bladder and urethra. Once Joellis started using the cream, her problems with urinary urgency and frequent urination went away.

Joellis's case is not unusual. After menopause a woman's level of the hormone estrogen lowers dramatically. Without sufficient estrogen, the tissue of the vagina and urethra areas becomes thinner and drier and may become weaker and more susceptible to irritation. This deficiency weakens the pelvic floor tissue and urethra and may result in atrophic vaginitis, a dry, red, and inflamed condition in a woman's vulva and urethral opening. Painful urination, burning sensations in the vaginal area, itching, frequent urination, painful intercourse, and urinary incontinence are indications of vaginitis. It is common for women to develop vaginal yeast infections, causing a white vaginal discharge that has a yeasty odor and a red rash in the perineum (the area around the rectum, vagina, and urethral opening). Estrogen cream or estrogen pills usually resolves associated temporary incontinence. If estrogen therapy is not an option, dietary supplementation with vitamins B complex (one tablet every day) and E (400 units daily) has been shown to be beneficial for certain women. Take these vitamins after a meal for maximum absorption.

MEDICATIONS CONTRIBUTE TO YOUR INCONTINENCE

No one knows what, if any, side effects you'll experience from taking a certain drug until you actually start using it. It's not uncommon for a person to take multiple medications, each prescribed by a different doctor who is unaware of what the other has ordered. Drug interactions can have serious consequences. It's in your best interest to know the name of each of your medicines, why it was prescribed, what are its most common side effects, how long you'll have to take it, if it is really necessary to treat your condition or illness, and how it interacts with other drugs you take.

If you look through any drug manual you will see incontinence listed as a possible side effect of hundreds, if not thousands, of registered drugs currently on the market. Incontinence among the elderly is often caused by prescribed drugs and overlooked by the doctors prescribing them. The older adult over the age of sixty-five takes on the average two to three drugs a day. The more drugs one takes, the greater the potential for side effects, including loss of bladder control.

DIURETICS

These are commonly called "water pills." They take excess water out of the bloodstream by increasing the amount of urine volume. Persons taking HCTZ (Dyazide) and furosemide (Lasix) may not have time to get to the bathroom before they leak. The time of day you take your diuretics is important. If you find you have to urinate several times during the night, take your water pill early in the morning. For example, if your dosage is two pills a day, take one at 6 A.M. and one at 2 P.M.

SEDATIVES, ANTIDEPRESSANTS, AND PAINKILLERS

These drugs dull the senses and may decrease a person's sensation of the need to urinate. If you've been given a sleeping pill, it is unlikely you'll consciously receive the message to go to the bathroom when your bladder is full. Sleeping pills and sedatives can cause an artificially deep sleep, masking the urge to urinate. They can make one feel groggy and disoriented on the way to the bathroom.

Good Advice

Remember, any medication, sedatives, pain killers, or antianxiety drugs that dull your brain, dull your bladder sensations.

These medications may also cause decreased bladder contractions, leading to incomplete bladder emptying. The bladder will not get the bladder urge message in time for you to get safely to the bathroom. Confusion and disorientation are also side effects of sedatives and you may not be alert enough to recognize your bladder's needs.

ANTIHISTAMINES, DECONGESTANTS, AND NASAL SPRAYS

These drugs (Antivert, Benadryl, Ornade, Sudafed, and so on) are prescribed to control allergies and allergic reactions to insect stings and certain foods. Side effects include sleepiness and drowsiness. These drugs may result in bladder retention and urine overflow because of bladder relaxation.

NARCOTICS

Narcotics deprive a person of clear sensory perception. You won't sense or feel the need to urinate. If you become constipated while using narcotics, excessive pressure is exerted on the bladder by the hard stool, decreasing its ability to hold urine.

ALCOHOL

Alcohol has a sedative effect that may alter a person's awareness of the need to void. Alcohol's diuretic effect causes the body to produce a larger volume of urine than you may be able to accommodate, causing incontinence.

THE HEALTHY MIND = CONTINENCE

A healthy and clear mind is important to maintaining continence. Confusion and depression can alter voiding habits and impede a person's recognition of bladder needs. Because coordination of messages between the nervous system and the urinary tract muscles and nerves begins in the brain, your mental state is a determining factor in the resolution of your incontinence.

ENVIRONMENTAL BARRIERS

Your living environment may contribute to your incontinence problems. Bathroom accessibility, hazards confronting you on the way to the toilet, and the condition of toilet facilities all affect you. Especially for the elderly, physical mobility or limitations present difficulties when using the toilet. By observing your toileting process, or how you use the bathroom facilities, a clinician can help you reduce the time it takes to use the toilet by yourself. When this "self-toilet" time is reduced, many regain their continence.

Physical disabilities brought on by a stroke, severe arthritis, or even an accident make using the toilet burdensome and, in some cases, nearly impossible. An environmental assessment of an incontinent person's home is an important part of a treatment plan. Equipment that enhances mobility such as canes, walkers, and wheelchairs should be available for persons who have ambulation problems. Individuals may be unable to reach the bathroom because of distance barriers such as furniture or other objects, poor lighting, or the need to climb stairs. The presence of a commode chair, bathroom grab bars, raised toilet seat, and toilet seat arms indicates that a home is, to borrow a computer term, "user friendly." Toilets must be at least 17 inches high with arms to assist the patient in lowering to or rising from the toilet seat.

Wheelchair patients find themselves in a special bind. Bathrooms in older homes and nursing homes and rest room facilities located in public buildings which were built before the Americans with Disabilities Act (ADA) was enacted are not always equipped to handle wheelchairs. Even though the ADA mandates that entrances, exits, and rest rooms must be handicapped accessible, many bathrooms and rest rooms are still reachable only by stairs, which, of course, can't be climbed when you're in a wheelchair. Wheelchair-bound individuals must be taught an easy method for using the toilet. When a bathroom is inaccessible or on another floor, a person can use equipment such as a bedside commode to regain continence. For those confined to a bed, male and female urinals, bedside commodes, and bedpans (commonly called collective devices) help maintain continence.

Physically restraining nursing home residents or homebound persons by using various straps and ties, as well as "geri-chairs" and chemical restraints such as sedating drugs, also increase the potential for UI.

There are other, more personal environmental factors. Clothing is, at times, a barrier to bathroom use. The amount of clothes or pads a person wears to protect themselves from urine leakage can hinder toilet accessibility. It is very hard for arthritic fingers to unzip pants. You can't lift your skirt or take down panty hose with a broken arm. How do you coordinate lifting up/pulling down clothes and steadying yourself on the toilet grab bars without something or someone falling? Adjusting clothing to make disrobing easier reduces a person's bathroom discomfort. Choose clothing that is easy to remove in the bathroom—wide, lift-up skirts, lapover skirts, and elastic or tie pants for women and men. As a rule, replace buttons at the waist with Velcro strips or snap closures.

Families, nursing homes, and public facilities must ensure that their bathroom and rest room facilities are conveniently located. The design should have easy access and use. Actually, this is not only for the benefit of incontinence sufferers; it is helpful for everyone who uses rest-room facilities.

CHAPTER 7

CHRONIC URINARY INCONTINENCE

Chronic urinary incontinence can be due to long-term changes in the bladder or urethra or is the result of damaged pelvic muscles and nerves. Chronic incontinence occurs because of persistent abnormalities of the structure or function of the lower urinary tract, including:

- Bladder overactivity—the bladder contracts when it should not.
- Bladder underactivity—the bladder fails to contract when or as well as it should.
- Urethral obstruction—usually due to an enlarged prostate or stricture (narrowing of the urethra).
- Urethral incompetence—the sphincter resistance is too low, resulting in urine leakage.

Chronic UI is classified into five types: stress incontinence, urge incontinence, overflow incontinence, functional incontinence, and reflex incontinence (see Table 7.1). In young adults each occurs alone, but mature adults and seniors may suffer from stress and urge incontinence, or mixed incontinence.

DO YOU HAVE SMALL LEAKS?: STRESS INCONTINENCE

Do you leak a small amount of urine when you cough, sneeze, or are physically active? Have you ever heard someone say "I laughed so hard I wet my pants"?

For the past eight months, Ruth, who is age thirty-eight, has noticed that her underwear is wet, or really just damp. It usually happens after she laughs or coughs hard. Recently Ruth started a new exercise program, and as the exercises have gotten more vigorous, her urine leakage has become more frequent. Ruth thought about stopping her exercise class, but she feels she can live with her problem. She wears a small panty liner, "just in case." When Ruth told her nurse friend Jane about her problem, Jane recommended that Ruth see a gynecologist. The gynecologist told Ruth that she had stress incontinence. Ruth told her doctor that she thought it might be related to stress because her five kids drive her crazy and "stress her out."

Ruth has stress incontinence, but it is unrelated to the psychological stress she associates with her children. Stress incontinence is related to pelvic floor support and increased pressure or stress on the bladder. The muscles in the pelvic floor area and the surrounding tissues are the key to urine control. As we learned in our discussion about the pelvic floor, weakened muscles and tissues in the bladder neck and the pelvic floor cause the bladder and urethra to sag or shift. Laughing, coughing, sneezing, running, jumping, exercising, lifting, sitting, standing, and strenuous physical activities cause a rise in abdominal pressure. As the stress, or pressure, increases, the bladder neck can't handle it—the pelvic support network isn't strong enough. The urethra can't control the flow of urine, and small bursts of urine leak out of the urethra. A damaged or weakened sphincter muscle might also be the source of leakage.

Typically, more women than men experience stress incontinence; six out of seven people with this problem are women. Because men don't have a uterus and don't carry and deliver babies, the pelvic muscles holding their organs in position are rarely stressed and stretched. Childbearing stretches and relaxes a woman's pelvic floor and may damage nerves in the pelvic area and tissue in the bladder's neck. Women sometimes talk of a "fallen uterus," one that has shifted within the abdominal cavity. The position of the uterus, bladder, and bladder neck within the abdomen has a direct effect on the control of urine. After menopause, a woman's estrogen level lowers, and it drops dramatically when the ovaries and uterus are removed during a hysterectomy. This further weakens pelvic floor and vaginal area muscles and tissues, increasing the likelihood of stress incontinence. Usually, women will try to cope with this problem by beginning a pattern of frequent urination; this is because a stress accident is more apt to happen with a full bladder. They may also complain that they lose urine when getting out of bed in the morning as the abdominal muscles push down on the bladder.

Stress incontinence occurs in men who've had prostate surgery and lost function in their urethral sphincter muscles. Excessive weight, constipation, or nerve injuries in the lower back can cause stress incontinence in both men and women.

Stress incontinence usually produces only small amounts of leakage. However, the severity of leakage may vary, depending on the specific activities that cause the urine loss. When leakage occurs only with relatively vigorous activities such as aerobics and coughing, laughing, and sneezing, it is termed minimal stress incontinence. Moderate stress UI occurs with less vigorous activities such as rising from a sitting to standing position or walking across a room. Severe stress UI occurs with minimal activity, such as changing positions in bed. Sometimes the leakage is not related to any activity. The signs and symptoms of stress UI are shown in Table 7.1.

Table 7.1 Summary of Types of UI

TYPES	SIGNS AND SYMPTOMS
Stress	Small amount of leakage of urine with increases in abdominal pressure—coughing, laughing, sneezing, physical activities, exercise
Urge	Unable to delay voiding after sensation of bladder fullness (urge) is perceived; moderate to large amounts of leakage, urine loss on way to bathroom, "key in lock" syndrome, urgency, frequent urination
Overflow	Bladder overfills until it finally overflows because an obstruction is preventing complete emptying, or muscle or nerve problems allow the bladder to overfill without giving the stimuli to empty; small, frequent voidings, postvoid dribbling, hesitancy, straining to void
Functional	Inability to reach bathroom because of loss of memory or because of physical disabilities that do not allow self-toileting.
Reflex	Loss of urine due to detrusor hyperreflexia and/or involuntary urethral relaxation in the absence of sensation usually associated with the desire to void

CAN'T ALWAYS MAKE IT THERE?: URGE INCONTINENCE

Never seem to make it to the bathroom in time?

Laura is very distressed. She never had any bladder control problems until she turned sixty-four, and now she can't control the urge to urinate. Sometimes the urge is so strong she feels she won't make it to the toilet in time if she doesn't run. The other day Laura really had an accident. Driving home from the mall, she got a strong bladder urge. She parked the car in the garage, grabbed her shopping bags, and rushed to the door. She fumbled with her keys, couldn't get them in the lock, and the urge was so strong that she completely "lost it." Laura wet through her pants. She was so glad she was home and not at the mall. Laura told her husband, who said that she probably has a

Table 7.2 Complex Diagnosis and Definition of Bladder Disorders

DIAGNOSIS	DEFINITION
Bladder (detrusor) sphincter dyssynergia (DSD)	Lack of coordination between the bladder and the pelvic floor muscles. Normally when a person attempts to empty the bladder, the pelvic floor muscles relax, allowing the urethra to open. Then the bladder contracts and pushes the urine through the urethra. With DSD, the pelvic floor muscles contract instead, clamping in on the urethra and interfering with the flow of urine.
Detrusor hyperreflexia (also called detrusor or bladder instability)	Hyperactivity or overactivity of the bladder muscle, caused by nerve impulses, often resulting in urge incontinence.
Type I stress incontinence	Mild stress incontinence when the bladder and urethra are in normal position; leakage only occurs with coughing, laughing, straining, and so on.
Type II stress incontinence	Moderate stress incontinence, in which leakage occurs with such activities as rising or walking.
Type III stress incontinence, Intrinsic urethral (sphincter) deficiency	Severe stress incontinence, in which the urethra does not work at all.
Atonic bladder	A bladder that is not able to contract and empty properly, usually because of damage to the nerves that control the bladder. As a result, the bladder fills with urine and remains full; excess urine that cannot fit in the bladder flows over and dribbles out through the urethra, causing overflow incontinence.
Detrusor with impaired bladder contractility (DHIC)	A condition characterized by involuntary detrusor contractions in which a person either is unable to empty the bladder completely or can empty the bladder completely only with straining, due to poor contractility of the detrusor.

weak bladder. Laura isn't sure whether she should mention her problem to her doctor, because all her friends seem to have weak bladders.

Laura has *urge incontinence*. Urge incontinence is the most common pattern of urinary incontinence in older persons. It is estimated that between 60 and 70 percent of seniors have urge incontinence. Urge incontinence is characterized by the "key in the lock" syndrome, such as Laura described. Other causes of leakage are running water when washing dishes or clothes, placing hands in warm water, anxiety, or exposure to cold. A person with this problem is very aware of the need to urinate and yet can't seem to get to the toilet before having an accident. Many complain that the urine just "gushes out." For all intents and purposes, the bathroom door might as well be locked tight, because the sufferer does not make it to the toilet in time to urinate.

In cases of urge incontinence, the bladder isn't properly controlling the urine release reflex. A detrusor muscle instability may impair the bladder's contractions, resulting in the immediate release of urine. The bladder does not have to be even close to full for a strong urge to be felt; sometimes just a few drops will stimulate bladder urge, contractions, and emptying. Or the bladder may be unstable due to infection or muscle and tissue damage. A person may have to strain to urinate and may retain urine. Tumors, stones, diverticulitis, Parkinson's disease, MS, strokes, and many other illnesses cause urge incontinence.

Mixed Incontinence

Most persons will have a combination of several types of incontinence called *mixed incontinence*. The most common pattern in older adults is a combination of stress and urge. However, a combination of overflow and urge is more common in men.

THE TANK DOESN'T EMPTY?:
OVERFLOW INCONTINENCE

Overflow incontinence occurs when there is blockage in the urethra or when the bladder can't properly contract.

People with overflow incontinence dribble small amounts of urine all day. They have difficulty starting the urine stream, and once started, the stream is weak. These individuals complain that they feel like their bladder never empties completely.

Ben who is sixty-eight years old noticed that his urine stream was slower and less forceful and never seemed to stop. Just when he thought he was done, some urine would dribble out and sometimes drip on the floor. Ben's wife was always complaining about the urine on the floor around the toilet. His doctor sent him to a urologist, who found that Ben's prostate was blocking the tube that carries the urine from his bladder. His urine dribbled because the tube had narrowed.

Ben has overflow incontinence. Overflow incontinence occurs when the urethra is narrowed or blocked by prolapsed (sagging or dropped) organs, a stricture, an enlarged prostate, or neurologic disease. When blockage is present, a full bladder can't empty and the urine just dribbles out. Because the bladder never gets to empty, it gradually stretches and stretches until it is unable to empty completely. People with overflow incontinence usually don't know they are leaking urine. Their sensation of a full bladder is diminished and their stream of urine is weak.

If overflow incontinence goes untreated, the bladder can become infected, sometimes leading to infection in the entire lower and upper urinary tract. In severe cases of overflow incontinence, the urine can back up into the kidneys, creating a dangerous medical problem. Blockage from an enlarged prostate gland is a common cause.

There are several causes of overflow incontinence. Diabetes and drugs such as narcotics, antidepressants, and smooth muscle relaxants may increase the capacity of the bladder, but they dull the sensation of the need to urinate. Trauma or injury to the spinal column nerves affects the urinary tract nervous system. Damaged bladder nerves and tissues reduce the bladder's ability to contract and release stored urine.

UNABLE TO GET TO THE BATHROOM?: FUNCTIONAL INCONTINENCE

In some cases persons experience urinary incontinence because they are unable to gain access to a bathroom.

Lucinda is eighty-two years old and lives in a row house in Philadelphia. Row houses are stately, old, narrow houses that are connected to each other. Her first floor has a living room, dining room, and kitchen. Bedrooms and the bathroom are on the second floor. In the morning, a nurse's aide comes to Lucinda's house to help get her bathed and dressed and downstairs. Lucinda spends most of her day sitting in her living room until her son comes at 6 P.M. to help her get ready for bed. When Lucinda has to use the bathroom, she has a hard time getting up her carpeted steps and is very fearful of falling. Many times she is incontinent before she reaches the bathroom.

Lucinda has *functional incontinence*. Functional incontinence involves a person's inability or unwillingness to use toilet facilities because of decreased mental awareness, loss of mobility, or personal reluctance to go to the toilet.

Over 25 percent of incontinence in patients in acute care hospitals and long-term care facilities is functional in origin. Even some hospitals have very poor and inconvenient bathroom facilities. Staffing problems, government and insurance companies' policies as to length of hospitalization, and medical treatment issues may place patient toileting habits low on the list of a hospital's priorities. Nursing homes may manage incontinence with protective products such as diapers. Individual patient needs and prior toileting habits are not usually part of the patient assessment process in long-term care facilities.

Common factors contributing to functional incontinence include:

- Restricted mobility or dexterity—inability or difficulty in getting to the bathroom or toileting because of physical disability.
- Environmental barriers—inconvenience of bathroom or toilet equipment, stairs, lack of handrails, narrow doorways which don't accommodate wheelchairs or walkers
- Mental and psychosocial disability—lack of awareness of the need to urinate, confusion over the location of the bathroom, or poor individual toileting habits
- Drugs—medications that affect awareness, mobility, or dexterity

Going to the toilet can be a real hassle. The elderly with impaired senses—poor eyesight, loss of hearing, difficulty in speaking—do not have the physical ability to reach and then use bathroom facilities. They might need help not only to get to the bathroom, but also with sitting down and getting up. Arthritic hands and fingers have trouble opening buttons and zippers. Clothes with snaps and elastic waists can be helpful to people with arthritis. Broken bones, dizziness, and painful joints also present barriers to using the bathroom. Then, too, if all of one's senses are not on the alert, communication is a problem. A person will have a hard time making caregivers understand what he or she needs, so may never get to do what is really wanted—to use the bathroom.

Environmental factors often accentuate immobility. The bathroom may be quite a distance away from a person's bed or chair. The route to the toilet may have steps, dark and narrow hallways, carpeted floors, and other obstacles. The door to the bathroom may be difficult to open and bathrooms with low toilets and no handrails are a real barrier for the elderly.

How can Lucinda be helped? Lucinda's daughter called the social worker at the nearby senior center and told her about Lucinda's fear of falling when walking to the bathroom. The social worker asked a continence nurse specialist to make a home visit to evaluate Lucinda and her environment. The nurse suggested that a bedside commode (portable toilet) be placed in the dining room or kitchen. The family and Lucinda had concerns about using a portable commode because of the need to empty the contents throughout the day. The nurse and the family decided that the best solution was to construct a small bathroom in the corner of the dining room. Once it was completed, Lucinda found she had no trouble getting to the toilet, and her fear of falling disappeared.

Mental confusion contributes to functional incontinence. A person may be completely unaware of the need to urinate. Memory plays tricks on everyone, and the elderly may forget where the bathroom is in their own homes and how to get to it.

HAVE NO FEELINGS TO URINATE?: REFLEX INCONTINENCE

Individuals with birth defects such as spinal bifida or spinal cord injury (paraplegics) do not have the urge sensation to urinate when the bladder contracts involuntarily. This is *reflex incontinence*. Many persons with this type of in-

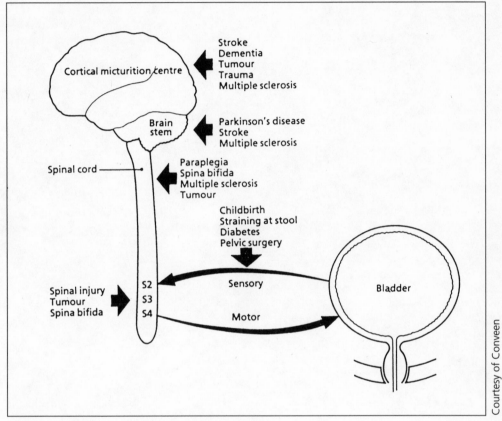

Figure 7.1 Possible neurogenic causes of incontinence

continence problem are diagnosed with a "neurogenic" bladder. (See Figure 7.1.) These individuals will have their bladders contract without the urge sensation to void, causing incontinence. Bladder evacuation will occur at unpredictable times and in response to volume or other stimuli such as cool air.

Damage to nerves in the spinal column, complications of surgery, and other spinal problems prevent the free flow of messages from the bladder to the brain and back to the bladder nervous system. When these bladder control center messages are disrupted, an individual has no indication of a full bladder. Reflex incontinence can be managed by toileting retraining and physical rehabilitation.

CHAPTER 8

RELATED CAUSES AND DISEASES

U rinary incontinence is not a disease or an illness. It is a symptom which occurs as the result of:

- A defined medical problem, including prostate disease, fecal incontinence, or diabetes.
- Part of a common bladder disorder called interstitial cystitis.
- A neurologic disorder which interferes with communication between the nerve pathways and the lower urinary tract and pelvic muscles, including multiple sclerosis (MS), stroke, Alzheimer's disease, diabetes, and Parkinson's disease.

Incontinence is not a normal result of aging, but older persons are more vulnerable to developing incontinence. Many elderly persons have illnesses that affect their remaining continence. The aging process, illness, or trauma can produce changes in the bladder control center in the brain. Neurological changes in the brain stem and spine can produce changes that give rise to poor coordination of bladder contraction and sphincter opening. (See Figure 7.1, page 69.) Also, many of the elderly with chronic illnesses are prescribed multiple medications that contribute or in many cases cause their urinaryincontinence.

LONG-TERM CHRONIC ILLNESS

A person with a spinal injury or a neurological disease, such as Alzheimer's disease, Parkinson's disease, or multiple sclerosis, has a lifelong struggle with bladder control. For wheelchair-bound individuals who wish to continue working, the discomfort and inconvenience of a bladder control problem present logistical nightmares that no one else can truly appreciate. Can others really understand the difficulties of trying to use a rest room while in a wheelchair or always looking for a clean and safe place in which to change a diaper?

ALZHEIMER'S DISEASE AND DEMENTIA

Dementia is characterized by mental deterioration. Dementia involves progressive lapses in memory, language, perception, learning, praxis (performance of daily activities), problem solving, abstract thinking, and judgment. Alzheimer's disease is a neurologic disorder in which certain memory, speech, intellectual, and muscular functions, including those of the bladder, deteriorate. Alzheimer's main characteristic is dementia. Dementia and Alzheimer's disease worsen over time. As these disorders progress, the affected person is completely unable to handle his or her personal care. Urinary incontinence occurs in the later stage of Alzheimer's disease because of changes in the part of the brain that affects urinary control. Persons with dementia should receive an assessment to ascertain acute or chronic causes of UI. Interventions include environment modification, toileting programs, and the use of appropriate devices and products to collect urine. Because of memory loss, individuals with Alzheimer's disease may not be aware of proper toileting habits. Many times the person will urinate in wastebaskets, closets, and flowerpots, as he or she cannot remember the appropriate place or bathroom location. Placing the word "toilet" on the door with a picture of the toilet at eye level is a great help. You should avoid interfering with the person when toileting, as any distraction is a barrier to urination. Traveling is a significant problem for a person with memory loss because a new toilet location is an overwhelming obstacle.

Two of the most successful interventions for continence maintenance for a person with dementia are adequate fluid intake and a toileting schedule. Individuals with Alzheimer's forget to drink fluids, particularly water. Reminding the individual to toilet every two to three hours is required. As the dementia progresses, the individual will have to be taken to the bathroom, require assistance with removal of clothing, and need to have verbal cues as to the toileting process. Instructions such as, "I want you to pull down your pants and underwear and sit down on the toilet so you can empty your bladder," may be necessary to achieve toileting. However, in the late stages of dementia and Alzheimer's disease, complete inability to control urination often occurs, and the individual usually has no recognition of incontinence episodes. At that time, the incontinence can only be contained by the use of products and devices (see Chapters 15 to 19).

STROKE

Stroke is a leading cause of severe disabilities. A stroke occurs when a blood vessel that feeds the brain gets clogged or bursts. The affected part of the brain can't work, and neither can the part of the body it controls. Stroke becomes more frequent with advancing age. Men are more likely to have strokes than women, and African Americans are more likely to have strokes than Caucasians. Urinary incontinence and other bladder dysfunction can occur after a stroke, usually within the first few days. Many individuals experience a lack of sensory awareness of the need to void or cannot control their bladders. Depending on the severity of the stroke and its effect on speech, many stroke victims are unable to communicate their toileting needs. Common bladder symptoms include frequency and urgency. Urinary retention may also occur, causing overflow incontinence.

A common bladder condition that occurs after a stroke is called uninhibited neurogenic bladder dysfunction. A person is able to sense the need to void and can start the stream, but cannot delay urination. Often the urge sensation is perceived when small amounts are present in the bladder.

A stroke can result in the person's inability to assist with being lifted, making his or her body heavier and feel like "dead weight." If an older woman is the caregiver, lifting a person who's had a stroke can injure her.

DIABETES

For persons over age sixty-five the classic symptoms of diabetes—excessive thirst, blurred vision, extreme hunger, dramatic weight loss, drowsiness, irritability, and mood swings—include two urinary symptoms, frequent urination and frequent urinary tract infections. As the diabetes progresses, persons may develop nerve damage. Sometimes nerve damage may interfere with the functioning of the bladder, and the bladder will not empty completely when one urinates. Persons with nerve damage as a result of diabetes have a reduced sensation to void.

RHEUMATOID ARTHRITIS

This is a general term referring to sore or swollen joints. Warning signs include swelling, redness, and pain at your joints; joint stiffness, especially in the morning; and restricted movement. Individuals with arthritis have mobility and dexterity problems that affect the ability to get to the toilet safely and in time.

PARKINSON'S DISEASE

Parkinson's disease is a degenerative disease of the nervous system characterized by tremor, rigidity, and bladder problems. Rigidity of muscles contributes to the inability to get to the bathroom and self-toilet. Muscle weakness affects the sphincter muscles, particularly the rectal sphincter, causing urinary and fecal incontinence.

Helen is eighty-three and lives with her sister. Helen was diagnosed with Parkinson's disease several years ago and has rapidly lost her physical functions. She recently moved in with her sister Patrice, who is several years younger. Lately, Helen has had increasing problems with urinary urgency and frequency, with occasional urinary incontinence episodes. Patrice has adapted well to Helen's frequent requests to go to the bathroom during the day, but during the night, this has become a great burden. Patrice reports waking up five to six times a night to toilet Helen and is starting to feel the strain. After several weeks of behavioral therapies, including bladder retraining with urge inhibition, pelvic muscle exercises, and fluid restriction after 6 P.M., Helen now has less UI episodes during the day, but there is no change at night. Patrice has always been resistant to using incontinence products, feeling Helen would become too dependent on them, but she has begun to realize that she can't last much longer on so little sleep. Helen and Patrice finally agreed on a plan of toileting during the day and incontinence products at night. After a month, the plan is working well for both of them.

Multiple Sclerosis

MS is a chronic disease of the nervous system characterized by fluctuating loss of muscular coordination and strength, as well as bladder problems. Urinary dysfunction occurs in about 80 percent of people who have MS. The loss of bladder control may be temporary, improving as the symptoms of the disease improve. However, most MS patients live with persistent urinary incontinence.

One of the most common causes of UI in persons with MS is a bladder infection.

Nicole is forty-six years old and was diagnosed with multiple sclerosis ten years ago. Nicole is worried that her husband will leave her if he learns about her accidents, both bladder and bowel. Nicole will feel humiliated if he finds out; he's been able to handle the MS, but Nicole isn't sure he'll handle this. Nicole's problem with bladder and bowel management has to do with urgency rather than full incontinence. She must make daily assessments as to her need for quick and easy availability of an accessible bathroom. Nicole has become somewhat physically disabled and needs to use a wheelchair. It takes more time for her to transfer from a chair or scooter to a commode. Nicole feels she's become obsessed with her disease and her needs.

For those with MS, a change somewhere in the central nervous system has interfered with the nerve signals from the spinal cord and the bladder control center in the brain. This causes a *neurogenic* bladder. One of the most significant bladder problems associated with MS is urinary retention—incomplete bladder emptying. In this case, the sphincter does not open properly when the bladder contracts, so the urine is not released. The person may be unaware that the bladder has not emptied completely by voiding. Instead, the person may experience urgency, frequency, nocturia (nightly voiding), and/or incontinence. Another cause of incontinence is that bladder contractions, which are involuntary, cause urination without control. In some patients the sphincter relaxes while the bladder contracts, allowing the patient to urinate normally but without control.

Initial treatments for urine loss due to MS include behavioral treatments—diet modification, bladder retraining, Kegel exercises, and medications (discussed in Chapter 15). If the bladder doesn't empty completely intermittent catheterization, discussed in Chapter 16, may be the solution. Management with incontinence products may be the only solution in cases of advanced MS.

Certain voiding maneuvers can improve bladder emptying in MS patients who have some component of neurogenic bladder with retention. They include the following:

- One technique to help stimulate complete bladder emptying is *trigger voiding*. The person who does not have any spinal cord injury may find a "trigger" to initiate a bladder contraction. A common method is called suprapubic tapping, which involves drumming the abdomen overlying the bladder. This tapping causes the bladder muscle to contract by activating the nerves. The best suprapubic triggering technique is to tap the suprapubic area rapidly seven or eight times, stop three seconds, and repeat. Other trigger mechanisms include pulling pubic hairs, stroking the abdomen or inner thigh, digital anal stimulation, and dilation. The clinician may want to experiment to discover which technique works best and most easily with each client.

- The *crede method* is a means of direct manual compression to empty the bladder. Press firmly with one hand (or both hands) directly into the abdomen over the bladder. Because bladder pressure is markedly increased, the bladder neck opens and emptying continues as long as the bladder is being compressed.
- A program of *double voiding* may be effective in cases of mild to moderate bladder obstruction. One must void twice during each trip to the bathroom to reduce residual urine volumes. The person voids, then voids again after a rest period of several minutes.

Interstitial Cystitis (IC)

IC is a bladder syndrome found mostly in women. It is a severe, debilitating, chronic disorder of the bladder. In the United States, IC affects approximately 500,000 persons, the majority of which are women. Persons with IC have a bladder wall that is tender and easily irritated, leading to uncomfortable symptoms. Women with IC complain of severe urinary urgency, frequent urination, lower abdominal or perineal pain and pressure, painful sexual intercourse, and, in many cases, urinary incontinence. IC begins gradually and may become progressively worse. Symptoms may go away for a while (remission), but may return.

Many persons with IC, especially women, are misdiagnosed. Women with chronic IC and severe nocturia may have depression due to sleep deprivation. Some doctors believe that IC has psychosomatic origins and tell women patients, "It's all in your head." This is not true. The exact origin of IC is not universally understood, but includes a variety of causes such as chronic infection of the bladder, lymphatic disease, autoimmune disorders (self-attacking diseases—the body turns on itself), and even psychologic and neurologic conditions.

Evaluating Your IC

You should see a urologist, who may be able to help you with your problem. Tests performed to diagnose IC are similar to the studies outlined in Chapter 10 and include urine cultures and urodynamic studies.

Treatment

Treatment for IC includes pharmacologic therapy, bladder stretching, and behavioral training. Bladder retraining and biofeedback (as described in Chapter 14) may be especially helpful to decrease symptoms of urgency and frequency.

Drug Therapy Some experts feel that IC is a chronic bladder infection problem caused by unusual forms of bacteria. Treatment requires several weeks of antibiotic therapy. Antibiotics used are Macrodantin and Augmentin. Medications such as analgesics and anti-inflammatory agents may be prescribed to decrease IC pain. Antidepressants in low doses may relieve IC symptoms by blocking pain receptors and relaxing the bladder muscle.

Behavioral Therapy In many IC individuals, pain and burning during urination happens because the pubococcygeus, or pelvic floor muscle group, is in spasm. Biofeedback therapy is helpful, especially in relieving IC flare-ups, as it teaches relaxation of the pelvic muscles. Electrical stimulation may help relieve symptoms by blocking the painful nerve signals to and from the bladder. It may also improve blood flow to the area and strengthen pelvic muscles. Bladder retraining is also successful in decreasing voiding frequency and urgency. It is important to compile complete bladder records so tracking of patterns and improvements can be monitored.

Dietary Modifications Changing your diet can help relieve and control symptoms and avoid flare-ups in the majority of IC cases. The idea behind changing your diet is to avoid foods that irritate your bladder. Following are dietary suggestions to help control IC.

This list of forbidden foods, noted in Table 8.1, may initially appear daunting; make adjustments by:

- Adding a pinch of salt to carbonated beverages to make them flat.
- Using reduced-acid orange juice now available in supermarkets.
- Boiling down all sauces containing alcohol.

Table 8.1 Dietary Suggestions

DON'TS	DO'S
Milk/Dairy Products aged cheeses, sour cream, yogurt, and chocolate	***Milk/Dairy Products*** white chocolate, nonaged cheeses such as cottage or American, frozen yogurt, and milk
Vegetables fava beans, lima beans, onions, tofu, spinach, and tomatoes	***Vegetables*** all other vegetables and home-grown, low-acid tomatoes
Fruits apples, apricots, avocados, bananas, cantaloupes, citrus fruits, cranberries, grapes, nectarines, peaches, pineapples, plums, pomegranates, rhubarb, strawberries, and juices made from these fruits	***Fruits*** melons, pears, and blackberries
Carbohydrates and Grains rye, sourdough, and pumpernickel bread	***Carbohydrates and Grains*** other breads, pasta, potatoes, and rice
Meats and Fish aged, canned, cured, processed, and smoked meats and fish, anchovies, caviar, chicken livers, corned beef, and meats which contain nitrates or nitrites	***Meats and Fish*** other poultry, fish, and meat

Many IC patients also have food allergies. The most common are wheat, corn, rye, oats, barley, and occasionally soy.

MANAGE YOUR STRESS Stress exacerbates IC symptoms or causes flare-ups. IC patients are advised to learn and practice basic relaxation techniques. Pain relief need not be provided solely by medication. Simple strategies which a patient can try at home include:

- Placing a cold pack, heating pad, or hot water directly on the perineum (area between the anus and vagina in women, and anus and base of

Table 8.1 Dietary Suggestions, *continued*

DON'TS	DO'S
Nuts	*Nuts*
most nuts	peanuts, almonds, cashews, and pine nuts
Beverages	*Beverages*
alcoholic beverages, beer, carbonated drinks, coffee and tea, and some herbal teas	bottled or spring water, decaffeinated, acid-free coffee and tea, and some herbal teas
Seasonings	*Seasonings*
mayonnaise, miso, spicy foods (especially ethnic foods such as Chinese, Indian, Mexican, and Thai), soy sauce, salad dressing, and vinegar	garlic and other seasonings
Preservatives and Additives	*Preservatives and Additives*
benzol alcohol, citric acid, monosodium glutamate, aspartame (Nutrasweet), saccharine, and foods containing preservatives and artificial ingredients and colors	
Miscellaneous	*Miscellaneous*
tobacco, caffeine, diet pills junk foods, recreational drugs, cold and allergy medications containing ephedrine or pseudoephedrine, and certain vitamins which may contain fillers	

penis in men). Experiment to determine if hot or cold works best
for you.

- Taking a warm "sitz" bath with or without Epsom salts. A sitz bath
  is a small plastic container that fits over the toilet and is available in
  drugstores.
- Placing your knees against your chest, reclining with spread legs, or
  adopting a squatting position.
- Practicing Kegel exercisings and focusing on completely relaxing your
  muscle between contractions.

ALLEVIATING PAINFUL SEX Sex can be a painful activity for women and men
with IC. Persons will avoid sex because they are afraid of urinary frequency,
pain, and discomfort. Others put up with painful sex because of worry about
rejection by their partners if the problem becomes an issue. Women report that
pain occurs because of lack of vaginal lubrication, from direct stimulation to
the clitoris, and during orgasm. Using lubricants (for example, vitamin E oil,
water-based gels, aloe vera gel) can ease pain during penetration. Having intercourse in different positions, such as with the woman on top or on her hands
and knees, will decrease clitoral stimulation and pain. Men with IC may have
difficulty with sex because of genital pain at the time of erection and frequent
need to urinate during sex. In these cases good communication with your partner is imperative. Avoid the use of latex condoms and the contraceptive diaphragm as these can cause IC symptoms.

BLADDER STRETCHING AND INSTILLATION In persons who have a low-
capacity bladder, stretching the bladder with fluid may bring temporary relief from symptoms. Sometimes filling the bladder with medication helps to
relieve inflammation and repair the bladder's irritated muscle. The medication is put in the bladder and retained for up to thirty minutes.

THERAPEUTIC MASSAGE Certain women, especially during an acute IC episode, benefit from applying ice and stretching the "trigger points" in the pelvic muscle. Trigger points are areas of hypersensitivity, and in IC persons, they can be found in areas such as the vagina, belly button, or upper thighs. Some women with IC will not wear belts or clothing with waistbands because they press on the trigger point in the belly button. Locating the trigger points along the piriformis muscle can assist in directing massage therapy. This muscle is found in the pelvis and upper thigh. The sacral and pudendal nerves exit the pelvis through the piriformis muscle. Another muscle that responds to ice massage is the abdominal muscle. Stroking the abdomen in overlapping vertical strokes from the rib cage to the pelvic bones will often relieve a woman's bladder pain. The goal with therapeutic massage is to reduce trigger points and reeducate muscles to regain their normal motion and function.

BOWEL AND FLUID MANAGEMENT Many individuals with IC are constipated due to pelvic muscle spasm and decreased fluid intake. Increasing fluids is an important part of IC management. Interventions to attain bowel regularity are outlined in Chapter 9 and can be used in cases of IC.

While there is still no cure, there are many treatments available. No single remedy works for every person, but the vast majority of IC problems can be brought under control by following the above recommendations.

MEN AND THEIR BLADDERS

Men can develop a variety of bladder disorders, all related to the prostate gland. The prostate is a walnut-size structure, present only in men. It surrounds the urethra like a doughnut. The gland secretes fluid that carries sperm during ejaculation. The gland becomes larger with age and hormonal changes, and by the age of sixty most men have an enlarged prostate. Disorders of the prostate include prostatitis, benign prostatic hyperplasia (BPH), and prostate cancer.

PROSTATITIS

This inflammation (swelling) of the prostate gland is caused by either a bacterial infection or by the backup of prostate secretions within the gland. Prostatitis may occur because of lack of sexual activity. Men with prostatitis have a small amount of watery discharge from the head of the penis, similar to a runny nose, and experience symptoms of frequent urination, discomfort when urinating, and urinary urgency. Infection or inflammation inside the prostate and urethra is usually caused by bacteria. Treatments include antibiotics, avoidance of caffeine, frequent ejaculations, no smoking, and increased fluid intake. If symptoms persist, bladder retraining and pelvic muscle exercises may be helpful.

BENIGN PROSTATIC HYPERPLASIA

In the young adult man, the healthy prostate is the size of a walnut. In the mid-forties the man's prostate may start to grow—enlarge on the inside—causing *benign prostatic hyperplasia* (BPH). BPH causes the prostate gland to enlarge, compressing the urethra and leading to partial obstruction of the urethra. The bladder muscle has to work harder to carry out its mission of emptying urine during voiding. Over time, as the bladder muscle enlarges, the overstretched bladder may contract weakly and with great difficulty or may be unable to contract at all. The bladder muscle loses function and can lead to detrusor instability. This results in frequent urination and nocturia. The first symptoms are:

- frequent urination—a feeling that you must urinate immediately
- nocturia—urinating at night
- hesitancy—a feeling of delay when you start to urinate
- a weak or interrupted urinary stream
- feeling that you are not emptying your bladder completely

In the past, the main treatment for BPH was transurethral resection of the prostate, surgery often referred to as a TUR or TURP (men often refer to this procedure as a "Roto-Rooter job"). In recent years the treatment of choice for BPH includes medication that relaxes the smooth muscle component of the prostate and less invasive surgeries that utilize new technologies such as lasers and thermal therapy.

PROSTATE CANCER

This is one of the most frequently occurring cancers in men, especially African American men. Today's cancer detection methods have increased the number of reported male prostate cancers through use of a blood test called PSA (prostate specific antigen). Unlike BPH, cancer of the prostate causes the prostate to enlarge on the *outside* of the gland. Unfortunately, symptoms of prostate cancer occur late in the disease. Another way to detect prostate cancer is through a digital rectal examination during which the physician can feel a nodule, or firm or hard area. The American Cancer Society recommends a digital rectal exam and PSA test annually in men over age forty. Symptoms of prostate cancer include a weak or interrupted stream of urine, inability to urinate, hesitancy, hematuria (blood in the urine), pain or burning on urination, and continuing pain in lower back, pelvis, or upper thighs. When prostate cancer is suspected because of an abnormal PSA or digital rectal examination, a prostate ultrasound and prostate biopsy must be considered.

There are several treatments for prostate cancer. The most popular is radical prostatectomy surgery (surgical removal of the prostate gland). Other treatments include radiation, hormone therapy, cryosurgery, and seed implants. Seed implants are radioactive needles left in the body to irradiate the cancer. Approximately 5 to 15 percent of men will experience urinary incontinence after prostate cancer surgery, especially in the first two to three months after the operation. This may be due to the fact that sphincter muscles in the urethra are weakened. Often UI is temporary, but sometimes it is a prolonged condition that causes anxiety and disruption in a man's life.

Treatment for postprostatectomy incontinence includes behavioral treatments, medications, urethral injections, or an artificial sphincter. Many men are shocked when they experience incontinence as a side effect of prostate surgery. They feel they were not informed that this could be a complication. Many are frustrated because the urologist who performed the surgery is disinterested in this side effect. Men need to know that there are treatments for UI, and they need to demand information and help from their doctors in seeking them.

Chapter 9

BOWEL IRREGULARITY

The control of urinary incontinence is linked to your bowels. The regularity or irregularity of your bowels affects your bladder and its ability to empty. Many people, especially as they age, tend to be "bowel obsessive." Every year, Americans spend $725 million on laxatives (drugs to make your bowels move). An integral part of an incontinence history includes a review of a person's bowels and his or her bowel habits. This chapter will discuss common problems that many persons with urinary incontinence experience: constipation, diarrhea, fecal impaction, and fecal (bowel) incontinence.

The large intestine is a hollow muscular tube about five feet in length. It is divided into the cecum, colon, and rectum. The cecum comprises the first two or three inches of the large intestine. The colon is subdivided into the ascending, transverse, descending, and sigmoid colon. The sigmoid colon bends toward the left as it joins the rectum, which allows gravity to aid the flow of water from the rectum into the sigmoid colon. (This is the rationale for lying on the left side when receiving an enema.) The last portion of the large intestine is the rectum, which extends from the sigmoid colon to the anus (about 6 inches). The last inch of the rectum is called the anal canal. It contains the internal and external regulating anal sphincters, which play an important role in controlling defecation. Muscle contractions in the colon push the stool toward the anus. By the time it reaches the rectum, it is solid because most of the water has been absorbed.

The nerve supply to the large intestine contains both parasympathetic and sympathetic nerves. In general, stimulation of the sympathetic fibers inhibits activity in the gastrointestinal (GI) tract. It also excites the internal anal sphincter. Thus, stimulation of the sympathetic fibers can totally block movement of food through the GI tract, both by inhibition of the bowel wall and closure of two major anal sphincters. Stimulation of the parasympathetic fibers causes an increase in bowel activity and in the defecation reflexes.

The large intestine has many functions, all related to the final processing of intestinal contents. Very little, if any, digestion takes place in the large intestine; its most important function is the absorption of water and electrolytes. Approximately 20 ounces of water is absorbed daily from the intestinal contents. The longer the fecal mass stays in the colon, the more water can be absorbed.

The movement of the intestinal contents in the large intestine is slow. Mass peristalsis, which is a contraction involving a large segment of the colon, moves the fecal mass into the sigmoid colon, where it is stored. This occurs two to three times per day, especially after breakfast.

Defecation is a reflex involving the muscles of the anal canal and large bowel. Entry of the fecal mass into the rectum distends the rectal walls and stimulates mass peristaltic movements of the bowel, which moves the feces toward the anus. As the fecal mass nears the anus, the internal anal sphincter contracts, and if the external anal sphincter is relaxed (under voluntary control), defecation will occur. The defecation reflex may be halted by voluntary contraction of the external anal sphincter. When this is done, the defecation reflex dies out after a few minutes and usually will not return for several hours. Water continues to be absorbed from the fecal mass, causing it to become firmer. This makes defecation more difficult and may lead to constipation.

Defecation is also facilitated by an increase in intra-abdominal pressure brought about by contraction of the chest muscles and simultaneous contraction of the abdominal muscles (Valsalva's maneuver, or straining).

CHRONIC CONSTIPATION

Constipation is usually considered the infrequent and difficult passage of stool, with fewer than three bowel movements per week. Usually, if more than three days pass without a bowel movement, the intestinal contents (stool) may harden or become pelletlike. A person may have difficulty or even pain during elimination and have to strain excessively to pass the stool. Older adults are five times more likely than younger adults to report problems with constipation. Older persons often become overly concerned with having a daily bowel movement and constipation may be imaginary. If the person also has urinary incontinence, once constipation is resolved, improvement in the number of "accidents" (episodes of incontinence) is seen. Constipation is a symptom, not a disease. But prolonged constipation can lead to urinary retention and incontinence.

Janet, sixty-six years old, came to my office complaining of leakage of urine with coughing, sneezing, and laughing. To try to decrease the severity of her incontinence, Janet limited her liquids. For the last five days, Janet noticed that she wasn't voiding that often and when she did void, there wasn't that much urine. She also noticed that her stomach felt bloated, and she was having a lot of gas and pelvic pressure. She was constipated one day last week, so she took Metamucil. The next day she had severe stomach pain but no bowel movement. Her pain went away. When I saw Janet, her stomach looked like she was six months pregnant, and her bladder was not emptying completely. She went home and started taking Milk of Magnesia. Once her bowels moved, she started voiding more frequently and larger amounts. Her bloating and pain went away.

Many persons have misconceptions concerning normal bowel habits. They feel that a bowel movement is necessary every day. Bowel patterns vary; having a bowel movement every other day or every third day may be normal. Also, some individuals feel that wastes in the bowel are absorbed and can shorten their lives. Therefore, these persons take large amounts and many different types of laxatives to have daily movements and to get rid of "harmful wastes." Heavy dependence on laxatives can become habit-forming. Their routine use interferes with normal functioning so that over time the bowels forget how to operate on their own. Plenty of other problems come with the habitual use of laxatives. Mineral oil coats the intestines and blocks absorption of vitamins A, D, E, and K and may also interact with other drugs you are taking. Milk of Magnesia pushes stool through your intestines so fast that nutrients are not completely absorbed. Chronic use of enemas leads to loss of normal bowel function.

Constipation is the result of many factors:

- Imbalanced Diet: A diet high in animal fats and refined sugars tends to be low in fiber. High-fiber diets result in larger stools, more frequent bowel movements, and less constipation.
- Poor Fluid Intake: Water and other fluids add bulk to stools, making bowel movements softer, more frequent, and easier to pass.
- Laxative Abuse: Individuals who habitually take laxatives become dependent upon them and may require increased dosages until the intestine becomes accustomed to the laxatives and does not respond to them properly.
- Travel: When traveling, individuals often experience constipation, especially during long-distances trips and travel to foreign countries.

This may be due to changes in drinking water, schedule, diet, and lifestyle.

- Hemorrhoids: Hemorrhoids are swollen veins in the anus or rectum. They can be *internal*, inside the rectum, or *external*, outside the anal opening. This condition causes pain, itching, and discomfort when passing stools and can cause spasms of the anal sphincter, delaying bowel movements. Hemorrhoid flare-up can be helped by drinking plenty of fluids, increasing diet fiber, and using witch hazel compresses. Surgery is an alternative in severe cases.

- Medications: Most of the medications commonly prescribed for older adults cause constipation. This is especially true with pain medications, antidepressants, antacids that contain aluminum, iron supplements, and tranquilizers.

- Diseases: Conditions such as multiple sclerosis, Parkinson's, stroke, and spinal cord injuries that affect nerves leading to the intestines or rectum and anus can cause constipation.

- Pregnancy: Women who are pregnant often have problems with constipation. This may be due to increased pressure from the baby on the intestines or hormonal changes.

- Lack of Exercise: A decrease in ambulation or prolonged bed rest due to an accident or illness may contribute to constipation.

- Restricting Fluids: Cutting down or limiting fluid intake can cause constipation.

CHILDREN AND CONSTIPATION

Constipation can be a problem for children and is usually due to poor bowel habits. Studies show that many who suffer from constipation as children continue to do so as adults. Children may hold their stools because of inconvenient toilets, difficulties at school, or emotional stress from a family crisis, causing constipation. Constipation in children may lead to fecal impaction.

Treatment

There are several different ways to treat constipation. The properly educated person can make the correct decision about which to use: laxatives, purgatives, and/or fiber. For most persons, dietary and lifestyle improvements can prevent constipation.

Fluids

Drinking plenty of fluids, preferably water, helps stimulate intestinal activity. Drinking a glass of prune juice daily or eating prunes may help with bowel regulation. Prune juice has almost no fiber, but does have a laxative effect, probably due to its content of magnesium salts. Prunes are relatively high in fiber (2 grams).

Fiber-Rich Foods

Foods rich in fiber help a person avoid constipation. Foods that have a high fiber content help to form bulky stools which pass more easily. High-fiber foods include:

- Whole grain breads and cereals (for example, All Bran); whole grain bread contains 8 to 10 percent dietary fiber, and some fiber-rich breakfast cereals contain 25 percent.

- Fresh fruits and vegetables, especially with the skin, are rich sources of fiber; they contain cellulose, hemicellulose, and lignin (lignin is not digested in the human intestine and therefore adds stool weight)—leafy green vegetables are especially good.

ADDING BRAN

One solution to constipation, if you can tolerate wheat products, is to use whole, unprocessed, coarse wheat bran, often called miller's bran. This is not the same type of bran found in widely advertised commercial bran cereals. Whole, unprocessed, coarse wheat bran can be purchased very inexpensively at health food stores and local grocery stores. The goal in using the bran is to produce one soft, well-formed bowel movement. You should begin using the bran in small amounts, such as 1 tablespoon, and gradually, over time, increase the amount you use. Bran can cause side effects—flatulence (gas), abdominal bloating, and cramps. But by starting out small and slowly increasing the amount, you can usually avoid these problems. However, if they do occur, they'll disappear in a few weeks. Sprinkle bran on your breakfast cereal and develop a routine of adding some bran to yogurt, Jell-O, cottage cheese, ice cream, or puddings. When cooking, put bran in sauces, muffins, gravies, and soups. Or make up a batch of the "special bran recipe" (see Table 9.2) and take some each day. Whole, unprocessed, coarse bran is safe for the body, and a person cannot take too much of it. In addition to using bran, drink at least six to eight glasses of caffeine-free liquids per day. Fluids aid bowel movements and also help stave off dehydration. For persons who are bedridden or are sedentary, the "special bran recipe" can be very helpful. The family can mix the recipe for the person. In nursing homes, the dietary department can make the recipe and give it to the nursing staff to administer to appropriate residents. It can be given in the same way laxatives are now dispensed.

Exercise

Physical exercise helps bowels stay regular. Get out for a walk or do some stretching, if you are not disabled.

Routine Bowel Schedule

In addition to taking fiber to regulate your bowels, it is helpful to maintain a routine schedule for moving your bowels. The optimal time is in the morning and after a meal. Sufficient time should be set aside to allow for undisturbed visits to the bathroom. In addition, the urge to have a bowel movement should not be ignored. This is especially important for residents in nursing homes who need assistance to toilet. If a regular toileting time is not set aside for the residents to empty their bowels, they will have bowel accidents. A bedridden person who lives at home or in a nursing home should try to avoid using a bedpan. Attempting to have a bowel movement on a bedpan is not natural. This posture causes undue strain if the person is not properly positioned. It forces the extension of legs, pushes the stomach (abdomen) out, and does not allow muscles to aid in defecation. Sitting upright allows gravity to assist in the passage of stool.

Mike is ninety-six and needs laxatives and sometimes even enemas to move his bowels. When he was young and active his bowels were regular, every day like clockwork. Once he stopped golfing five years ago, he noticed a change. If his bowels don't move for two days he takes Milk of Magnesia. If they still don't move, he takes Dulcolax tablets and sometimes even mineral oil. He may go four days without having a bowel movement, and his wife has to give him an enema. His doctor knows about his problem and sent Mike to a nurse practitioner who specializes in bowel problems. She gave Mike a bowel schedule. He was told to sit on the toilet every morning after break-fast, since meals (especially warm food or drinks) stimulate the bowels to move. Mike was to raise his feet on a footstool when he sat on the toilet be-cause this position aids in bowel evacuation. If his stool is hard, Mike was told to put a glycerin suppository in his rectum. Mike was also told to take the "special bran recipe." After three weeks of following these instructions, Mike saw a big difference. He was having a bowel movement almost every day on schedule after breakfast. He only had to use a suppository a couple of times a week. However, the bran did give him flatulence (gas).

Mike was successful in improving his bowel function. You can be, too. What should Mike do about the gas? Some foods contain starches that es-cape digestion in the small bowel and may cause gas in the colon. A list of foods commonly thought to cause gas follows. Try cutting these foods out of your diet and see if you have less gas, or just wait a few weeks to see if your body adjusts to the higher fiber.

Apricots	Lentils
Bananas	Milk and milk products
Beans	Onions
Brussels sprouts	Peas
Cabbage	Pretzels
Carrots	Prunes
Celery	Raisins
Dried beans	Wheat germ

If for some reason you need to use laxatives, suppositories, or enemas you should become knowledgeable about what you are using. Table 9.1 will help educate you about the various products available.

Tips for Preventing Constipation

Prevention is the best approach to most bowel problems and can be successful in keeping your bowels regular. To prevent constipation:

- Identify your normal bowel habits and do not rely on laxatives.
- Eat a well-balanced diet, including grains, fruits, and vegetables, and add unprocessed bran.
- Drink plenty of water.

Table 9.1

TYPE OF PRODUCT	ACTION	EXAMPLES
Stool softeners	Provide moisture to the stool and prevent excessive loss of water. Often recommended after surgery and childbirth. Effective within 24 to 48 hours to produce firm, semisolid stool.	Dioctyl sodium succinate (Colace, Pericolace)
Lubricants	Grease the stool, allowing it to slip through the intestine more easily. Effects are usually noted within 6 to 8 hours.	Mineral oil
Bulk-forming agents	Absorb water in the intestine to make stool softer; should be taken with 8 ounces of water. Safest laxatives but can interfere with absorption of some drugs. Takes 12 hours to 3 days to be effective.	Bran, psyllium (FiberCon), methylcellulose (Metamucil, Citrucel)

- Exercise regularly even if it is walking in the mall or walking your dog.
- Allow for scheduled time (20 to 30 minutes) after breakfast or dinner to have an undisturbed bowel movement.
- Never ignore your urge to defecate.

DIARRHEA

Most individuals will have an occasional episode of diarrhea, lasting maybe one or two days. Diarrhea is the passage of frequent, watery bowel movements.

Table 9.1, continued

TYPE OF PRODUCT	ACTION	EXAMPLES
Osmotic cathartics	Cause water to remain in the intestine for easier movement of stool. Produces watery stool in 3 to 6 hours.	Milk of Magnesia, magnesium sulfate or citrate, lactulose
Stimulants or irritants	Cause rhythmic muscular contractions in the intestines. These can cause dependency, and can damage bowel with continual use. Effects are usually noted within 6 to 10 hours.	Cascara, castor oil, senna (Senokot, Fletcher's Castoria), Bisacodyl (Dulcolax), phenolphthalein (Correctol, Ex-Lax)
Enemas	Instill fluid into the rectum for removal of stool.	Tap water, saline, sodium phosphate (Fleets), milk and molasses
Suppositories	Trigger the defecation reflex and assist the rectum to empty any stool contents.	Oil, glycerin, bisacodyl (Dulcolax)

Table 9.2 Special Bran Recipe

If you are constipated, the following recipe will help you.

Mix together:

> 1 cup applesauce
> 1 cup coarse unprocessed wheat bran
> ¾ cup prune juice

This mixture should have a pasty consistency. Refrigerate in a covered container between uses.

**HOW OFTEN DO I EAT
THE SPECIAL RECIPE?**

Begin with 2 tablespoons of the mixture every day with a glass of water. Take the mixture in the evening for a morning bowel movement. Increase the quantity you take by 2 tablespoons each week until your bowel movements are regular. Always drink one large glass of water with the mixture.

**WHAT IF I DON'T LIKE
THE SPECIAL BRAN RECIPE?**

Just add unprocessed wheat bran to your diet. Start by using 1 to 2 tablespoons every day. If necessary for regulation, increase bran slowly over several weeks to approximately 6 tablespoons every day.

**HOW TO ADD BRAN
TO YOUR DIET**

Keep bran in a bowl or shaker on the table and sprinkle it on ice cream, vegetable and fruit salads, or cottage cheese. Cook with bran and add to muffins, breads, and cookies when baking or in foods like applesauce, cereals, sauces, gravies, or puddings.

**WILL BRAN
HARM ME?**

NO! The normal reaction to bran is stomach bloating and increased gas. These symptoms usually last for only the first week. If symptoms last longer, contact your nurse or doctor immediately.

Good Advice

To help you have regular bowel movements, follow these steps:

Step 1 Try to have a bowel movement in a private place and after a meal, such as breakfast. Both eating and the smell of appetizing foods can cause your bowels to move.

Step 2 Drink something warm with your breakfast, such as warm water. This will also help the bowels to move.

Step 3 Twenty minutes after eating breakfast, sit on the toilet or bedside commode.

Step 4 Put your feet up on a footstool and push your body forward a little while on the commode.

Step 5 Massage or rub your lower stomach to push the bowel movement into your rectum.

Step 6 Have patience—it may take twenty to thirty minutes for you to have a bowel movement.

Step 7 Use glycerin or Dulcolax suppositories, if necessary, to make it easier to move your bowels. Insert a bisacodyl or glycerine suppository in your rectum within one hour before breakfast. Place the suppository against the rectum wall and administer daily until a consistent bowel pattern is identified.

Step 8 Put a lubricated (with K-Y Jelly) finger in your rectum, if necessary, to help your bowels move. Be sure to wash hands before and after doing this.

The symptoms disappear quickly and are more an inconvenience than an illness. But in certain cases, diarrhea may persist for days, weeks, and even months and may be caused by a major disorder. If this occurs, you may have viral or bacterial diarrhea due to the flu, a virus, or food poisoning. Diarrhea can be caused by an infectious process and raises particular concern in institutional settings, such as hospitals or nursing homes, where an infection may spread among the resident population. The *Clostridium difficile* bacteria, which causes

diarrhea, is usually treated effectively with medications. Another cause of diarrhea, especially in
the older adult, is laxative abuse. Regular, frequent
use of laxatives disrupts the nerves to the colon,
dulling the sensation for bowel elimination. Natural emptying mechanisms fail to work as the body
becomes dependent on laxatives and enemas.

> **Good Advice**
>
> If you have prolonged
> diarrhea, an impacted
> bowel problem that you
> can't resolve, or both uri-
> nary and fecal inconti-
> nence, see your doctor!

Symptoms such as abdominal cramping, frequent passage of thin, watery stools,
change in color and odor of stool, nausea and vomiting, and even fever may
occur. If your doctor feels that your diarrhea is caused by an infection, he or
she may wish to test your stool for bacteria. This test is called a stool culture.
Prolonged diarrhea can cause skin irritation and breakdown around your anal
area. You should clean this area after each movement with mild soap and water, pat it dry, and apply petroleum jelly or some type of cream. Good skin
care protects the skin and helps relieve discomfort.

TREATMENT

- Add fiber to your diet; this will add bulk to decrease the amount and
  frequency of watery liquid. Fiber's function is to bind with water in
  the intestine to form a gel. This prevents its overabsorption from the
  large bowel and insures that the fecal content of the large bowel is
  both bulky and soft.
- Avoid eating foods that contain caffeine (tea, coffee, chocolate, soft
  drinks). Caffeine consumption causes increased fluid secretion in the
  intestine, thus increasing the amount of diarrhea.
- Talk with your doctor or nurse about the medications you are taking.
  Some cause diarrhea; for example, antacids containing magnesium
  and antibiotics.

FECAL IMPACTION

Fecal impaction is stool that has built up over several days and hardened in your rectum (see Figure 9.1). Fecal impaction is not very common, but it may occur in frail, ill older persons or in children with neurologic diseases. If it

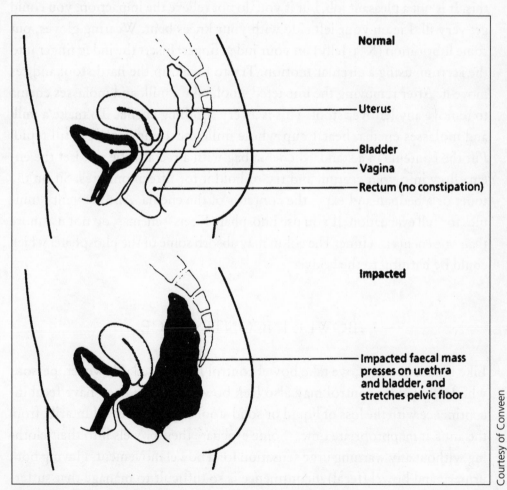

Figure 9.1 How constipation can cause urinary incontinence

occurs, you are usually unable to pass this large amount of stool. You may pass small amounts of watery stool and experience severe stomach pain, discomfort, and bloating. You may lose your appetite. Some very ill older persons may also have a change in behavior and have a fever. If a large impaction is present, it may need to be broken up manually, using your fingers. You should have a family member or someone close to you assist you in doing this. It is not a pleasant job, but if you do not relieve the impaction, you could get very ill. Lie on your left side with your knees bent. Wearing gloves, put some lubrication (K-Y Jelly) on your index finger. Insert the index finger into the rectum, using a circular motion. Try to break up the hard stool and remove it. After removing the impacted stool, take a milk and molasses enema to remove any leftover stool. This is a very soothing enema. To make a milk and molasses enema, heat 1 cup whole milk and 1 cup molasses till tepid. Put the contents in a standard enema bag with a rectal-tube tip. Let the enema flow into your rectum and try to hold it for fifteen minutes. Sit on the toilet or a bedpan and expel the contents of the enema. Allow twenty minutes for full evacuation. If you use phosphate Fleets® enemas, do not use more than one enema at a time. The colon may absorb some of the phosphate, which could be harmful to the body.

BOWEL INCONTINENCE

Like bladder control, we take bowel control for granted. However, persons who lack bladder control may also lack bowel control. They have fecal incontinence with the loss of liquid or solid stool or pass gas involuntarily from the anus at inappropriate times. Some evacuate their bowels into their clothing without any warning urge sensation for a bowel movement. Having both urinary and bowel (fecal) incontinence is so difficult to manage that sufferers live in a constant state of anxiety and may totally withdraw from society.

The reason both types of incontinence may occur at the same time is that the digestive tract and the lower urinary tract are closely connected, and anything that affects one can affect the other. Both systems share common nerves and both are supported by the pelvic muscles and other structures that play a vital role in maintaining continence. As mentioned in Chapter 2, the nerves of both the urinary tract and the digestive tract arise from a common source, the pudendal nerve. Therefore, anything that cuts or damages this nerve source will cause urinary and fecal incontinence. Diseases or injuries which affect the spinal cord or the nerves or muscles can affect both systems. In adults, the most common cause of fecal incontinence is obstetric or the result of surgical trauma, usually a direct injury to either the anal sphincter or the pudendal nerve. Rectal sensation warns of imminent defecation and helps you discriminate between formed and unformed stool and gas. Impaired rectal sensation may deprive a person of this useful information and result in incontinence.

Since the nerve branches of the urinary and digestive system come off the same trunk, it is possible to handle both kinds of incontinence with a single treatment. Therefore, a person receiving biofeedback treatment as a therapy for urinary incontinence may be taught to use biofeedback to contract his or her anal sphincter. Pelvic (Kegel) exercises, which involve tightening the pelvic floor muscles, are also very useful for learning to tighten the anal sphincter.

Among older people, the most common cause of fecal incontinence is neither loss of mobility or dementia, but simply the natural effects of aging on the body. Muscles and tissues weaken, lose their elasticity, and become lax. Changes in muscle strength, muscle mass, and muscle and nerve reflexes affect the rectum and anus just as they affect our arms and legs. Thus, some older people can't retain gas or stool, especially liquid stool, as well as or for as long as they once could. Also, the older person may not be able to reflexively close the anal sphincter quickly enough to avoid a fecal accident. Compared to continent people, incontinent elderly people have less rectal sensation and less sphincter strength.

Severe constipation can make you have bowel incontinence. The constipation can lead to a large amount of stool in the rectum, or fecal impaction, discussed earlier. The impaction interferes with your normal ability to control your bowel movements. A liquid stool eventually trickles around the impaction and leaks out.

As with any other medical problem, understanding the cause of your bowel incontinence is important. Bowel and urinary incontinence are very similar in that they are hidden problems, causing social isolation and dysfunction.

CHAPTER 10

FINDING HELP FOR
YOUR INCONTINENCE

Joyce started leaking small amounts of urine around the time she stopped menstruating thirty years ago. As she was experiencing other symptoms of menopause (night sweats, headaches), she didn't become concerned about the incontinence. Urine loss only happened maybe once a week and only when she was rushing and wasn't careful. It was a nuisance, but she managed. About a year ago, she started to notice that the urine leakage was occurring more often, maybe twice a week, and there didn't seem to be a reason for it. Joyce mentioned it to her gynecologist, who told her it was common. He didn't suggest what she should do, but then Joyce didn't really ask.

Surveys show that two-thirds of people suffering incontinence are dissatisfied with their treatment. Men will seek treatment after a year and a half, whereas women wait three and a half years. The biggest complaint patients have when they consult a health care professional about their urinary incontinence is that they are not advised about the wide range of treatment possibilities. A Harvard University Medical School study reported that when patients do mention incontinence, fewer than one in three doctors will initiate even the most basic evaluation.

Karen has been losing urine for years, especially on the way to the bathroom. Karen is a woman who seeks solutions to problems, and her incontinence is a problem. She saw a urologist ten years ago and his diagnosis was "poor hygiene." Karen is only seventy-two years old, and she is still looking for a solution to her incontinence.

Why is this? Most doctors and nurses view incontinence as an inevitable part of aging. The subject has been neglected in medical schools, with very little hands-on training in managing the problem. Traditionally, incontinence has been a nursing care problem. Unfortunately, to some nurses, managing incontinence means putting a patient in a diaper or using a catheter. Even urologists, who are the incontinence specialists, find incontinent patients uninteresting and cumbersome unless the problem can be surgically "cured." The amount of time it takes to listen to the toileting behavior and care procedures of someone with incontinence is not profitable. Medicare and most insurers do not value the teaching time it takes to review and identify behavior and habits and to attempt to apply effective solutions and approaches.

Today, however, more persons are consulting professionals who are in the business of treating incontinence. Medical and nursing schools now offer health care students courses with incontinence content. The American Nurses Association has issued competency guidelines on urinary incontinence nursing assessment and treatment for baccalaureate and graduate-level nurses.

Incontinence care and management is a growing and expanding health care field. Insurers, even HMOs, understand that UI is a hidden problem that needs to be addressed once it is identified. There is a growing understanding among physicians, nurses, and other providers that there are several treatment options open to men and women with UI. It is important for the consumer to understand that if you suffer from urinary incontinence, you should seek help or find a resource person. The problem will not go away; it will slowly get worse as you age. To locate a resource person call your local hospital, home health care dealer, or local pharmacy, or ask family and friends. This chapter will outline the various providers in the health care field who are able to help you with your problem.

THE FIRST LINE OF DEFENSE

Your family doctor is your first line of defense when seeking help for an incontinence condition. Family doctors are usually general practitioners or internists and most have knowledge of the dynamics of UI. If they cannot help solve your UI, you may be referred to a specialist. Alternatively, you may decide on your own to initially visit a UI specialist.

CHECKING OUT PRACTITIONERS

Always check out a new professional before your first visit. Experience, expertise, and reputation indicate a professional's competence whether he or she is doctor or a nurse. Family, friends, and colleagues are good sources of information about competent incontinence providers. Your local medical society doesn't rate doctors, but usually will provide a list of specialists.

Before your visit, investigate:

Good Advice

If your doctor disregards a urinary incontinence problem, treats it as a normal part of aging or something you just have to live with, and does not investigate the underlying cause, find another doctor!

- Training—What schools did the provider attend? Did the provider take special training for incontinence treatment?
- Practice—Is the provider a solo practitioner? Does the practice employ clinicians and technicians trained in incontinence treatment? If

the provider is in a partnership, does every member of the practice have expertise and experience in diagnosing and treating incontinence? Are members of the practice available to help patients as needed?

- Certification—Has the provider taken some type of board specialty exam in a related field? At this time, there is not an incontinence specialty test for doctors.
- Clientele—What percentage of the provider's client load is devoted to incontinence treatment? What is the success rate for incontinence treatment? A measure of success is how dry they get their patients.
- Affiliations—Is the provider affiliated with any hospitals? At which local hospitals does the provider have staff privileges? Is the provider affiliated with any nursing homes or long-term care facilities?
- Is the provider familiar with urodynamic testing, biofeedback therapy, exercise, and other incontinence treatments? Do they provide these services?
- Will the provider accept your insurance?

THE PHYSICIAN

Medical doctors who work with persons with incontinence should be familiar with the various types of incontinence, available and proven treatments, and urodynamic testing. You may first choose to go to a family physician, or you may go to a specialist. Unfortunately, in this age of managed care and HMOs, you may not have the opportunity to develop a close relationship with your primary care or family doctor. HMO primary care physicians may not see the need to refer a person to a specialist. HMO and managed care insurers readily refer a person for incontinence surgery, but do not cover behavioral services such as biofeedback therapy. Older adults, who are Medicare patients, may also have little choice in selecting their physicians.

There are several types of physicians who are qualified to handle the problem of urinary incontinence.

FAMILY DOCTORS

You have a unique relationship with your family doctor, who is usually a general practitioner or an internist and your primary care physician. You've probably known and visited this doctor over a period of time. This long-term relationship provides an atmosphere in which to comfortably discuss your incontinence. Having treated your routine illnesses, your family doctor maintains your medical history—a record of your illnesses, prescriptions, tests, and surgeries. In many cases, after a discussion of your symptoms, an examination, and possibly some tests, the family doctor can help you design a treatment plan for your incontinence. However, if you need special help due to conditions such as cancer, an enlarged prostate, or a urinary tract infection, you'll be referred to a specialist.

GERIATRICIANS

These physicians offer care and treatment for older adults and the elderly. They are particularly experienced in handling the relationship between aging, medication use, and bladder changes.

GYNECOLOGISTS

This group of doctors treat conditions of the urinary and reproductive system in women. They are usually the primary physicians for dealing with pelvic area problems. They perform hysterectomies and bladder neck surgery, and also deliver babies. At your yearly exam, your gynecologist should ask you if you have any bladder problems or any urinary symptoms that interfere with your lifestyle. A relatively new specialist, the urogynecologist, has emerged from this group. These are surgeons who treat problems of the bladder and uterus in women.

UROLOGISTS

These surgeons treat bladder and urinary tract difficulties and incontinence conditions. They are also specialists in the area of prostate gland problems and the male reproductive system.

THE NURSES

Taking care of incontinence is a basic part of nursing practice. Nurses care for patients in all age groups and their practices span all types of medical settings. Nurses are professionals—either registered nurses (RN) or licensed practical nurses (LPN).

NURSE PRACTITIONERS

These professionals include advanced practice nurses and clinical nurse specialists with postgraduate education; they can work as independent practitioners. Many nurse practitioners have developed a specialty in the area of incontinence evaluation and treatment. Their expertise includes the management of chronic "intractable" incontinence, which is incontinence that has not responded to treatment with medications, surgery, and behavioral training. They provide urodynamic testing, Kegel exercises training, biofeedback therapy, bladder retraining, and other services, particularly management through the use of catheters, products, and devices. In most states, nurse practitioners can prescribe medication and other treatments and many are in independent practice and work in conjunction with physicians.

Enterostomal Therapy Nurses (ET)

ET nurses provide ostomy (an opening in the gastrointestinal canal), wound, and incontinence care. They are specialists in the care of skin problems, and many are involved in the assessment, evaluation, and care of incontinent persons.

Rehabilitation Nurses

Rehab nurses work with individuals who have suffered medical events which have impaired their physical functions. Heart attacks, strokes, and spinal cord injuries are among the events which may cause incontinence. These nurses are trained to help patients regain as much of their physical functions as possible.

Nursing Aide

The aide plays an invaluable part in the care of persons with incontinence, especially in hospitals, home care, and nursing homes. They are skilled in assisting with patient personal hygiene, toileting, and helping families learn toileting programs and manage incontinence.

THE THERAPISTS

Physical therapists (PT) and occupational therapists (OT) are really physical retrainers. Physical therapists assist in helping the person gain lower leg and upper body strength, increasing mobility and balance and making it possible to get to the toilet in a safe and quick manner. They are excellent teachers of safe and effective transfer techniques for caregivers. PTs teach pelvic muscle exercise reeducation. Occupational therapists can evaluate the environment in and around the toilet area and provide assistive devices for the toilet such as handles and a raised toilet seat. They evaluate clothing and dressing techniques, offering ideas regarding easier ways to manage clothing. OTs also work with a person's memory problems to assist with toileting behaviors. Speech and language pathologists have training in communication skills and cognition disorders and are very helpful for persons with dementia and urinary incontinence.

THE SOCIAL WORKER

Social workers help you deal with the social and financial concerns of your problem, especially if you are caring for a family member with UI. They have a vast knowledge of available local community, state, and federal programs that provide services and financial support to assist with incontinence care. Social workers are trained counselors and have the tools to effectively help the incontinent person work through feelings of depression, embarrassment, or isolation. In many cases, social workers are case managers who provide overall supervision for persons with complex medical problems.

THE PHARMACIST

Pharmacists play a role in patient assessment, intervention, and education. Some pharmacists consult with nursing homes and deal with urinary incontinence on a daily basis. The retail pharmacist has an important function as a front-line health professional who can interact with ambulatory individuals who visit the pharmacy to purchase incontinence medications, supplies, and products. The pharmacist is an invaluable resource for the person seeking answers to control UI, providing drug therapy education to consumers, and ensuring that each medication's purpose and importance are understood.

MEDICAL PRODUCT SUPPLIERS

A medical product supplier may be your local drugstore, a home health care dealer, a DME (dealer of medical equipment), or a mail-order catalog supplier (see Appendix A). All these types of businesses provide you with the supplies, products, and equipment needed to manage your incontinence. Even the Sears catalog contains medical products. However, be careful what you purchase. Products should only be used after your problem is evaluated by a doctor or nurse. Chapters 16 to 19 will give you information on the proper use and care of these products.

INCONTINENCE PRACTICES

Over the past decade, incontinence specialty practices have sprung up across the United States. Typically, they are headed by physicians, urologists or urogynecologists, and/or nurse practitioners. Clinicians in these practices provide physical, vaginal, and rectal examinations, pelvic tissue and muscle examination, urinalysis, and urodynamic testing. Up-to-date treatment plans—behavioral therapy, biofeedback, electrical stimulation, and bladder retraining—are offered in these practices. Incontinence practice clinicians are in the forefront of raising public awareness about incontinence and educating the public about UI treatment therapies. The author has had such a practice, Access to Continence Care & Treatment, in the Philadelphia area for the past ten years. It is unique because of its emphasis solely on urinary incontinence and related problems. The practice provides office services, in-home care, and nursing home care.

The National Association for Continence has a list of continence experts. Call 1-800-BLADDER to get the name of a provider in your geographical area.

Chapter 11

YOU CAN RUN,
BUT YOU CAN'T HIDE

If you have urinary incontinence you probably aren't objective about your condition. Feelings of shame, humiliation, and confusion frequently accompany the condition, clouding decisions. As we've noted, by attempting to hide incontinence from doctors, nurses, family, and friends, incontinence sufferers place themselves in a position of never accessing the help that is available. Or they dismiss their condition, but reluctantly admit, "I have some problems with my bladder." However, as the problem worsens, as it undoubtedly will without treatment, it becomes difficult to conceal. Sadly, this "conspiracy of silence" can cause more shame than the incontinence.

INVESTIGATING THE CAUSES

An objective determination of the problem is the first and most important part of the evaluation and treatment of incontinence. Symptoms of bladder and urinary tract problems may indicate the presence of incontinence, but again they may not. Neither do they always provide clues as to the possible cause of the problem. That is why the assessment of an incontinence problem should be referred to a competent clinician who has experience in the diagnosis and treatment of incontinence.

IDENTIFYING YOUR SYMPTOMS

Treatment of UI depends on the type of incontinence, severity, and medical condition. Your medical history is the cornerstone of the diagnosis of your problem. The physical examination and test results must be correlated to your history in assessing your urinary situation.

> **Good Advice**
>
> **W**rite down your symptoms, problems, and questions before you visit the doctor. That way, you won't forget anything important during your examination.

The doctor should thoroughly and carefully question you about your symptoms and urinary habits. Be certain to describe all of your problems in detail. Make a list of your symptoms and take it with you to your doctor.

For instance, you might be experiencing lower abdominal pain. On the other hand, if the problem is related to some type of neurologic injury, you may have little or no pain. Make a note on your list about your pains or lack of them. The information will aid in the diagnosis of your condition. If your physical condition prevents you from writing out the list on your own, ask a family member, a friend, or your nurse for help in compiling your list. The clinician will want to rule out any reversible or acute causes of incontinence, as detailed in Chapter 6.

WHAT? WHERE? WHEN? HOW?

Based on the description of your problem and the pattern of incontinence, the characteristics—onset, frequency, and severity—will be noted and evaluated when you visit a clinician, who is either a doctor or a nurse.

Before you visit a clinician, you should make some determinations about the type of incontinence you have. Ask yourself:

- Do you ever leak urine when you don't want to do so?
- How often do you go to the bathroom?
- Do you lose or leak urine when you laugh, cough, sneeze, lift heavy objects, walk, or sleep?
- Do you leak urine when you work out or do aerobics?
- Do you always go to the bathroom when you're near one, just in case?
- Do you constantly go to the bathroom because you're afraid of wetting yourself?
- Do you lose urine on your way to the bathroom?
- Does the urge develop abruptly?
- Do you dribble urine after you void (urinate)?
- How long can you comfortably go between urinating?
- Do you wake up from sleep wet or to go to the bathroom?
- Have you lost urine during or after sex? During your periods? During pregnancy or after childbirth? At the onset of menopause?
- Do you lose urine at the sound, sight, or feel of running water?
- Do you use pads or diapers to collect your urine?
- Do you have difficulty starting your urine flow?
- How often do you urinate?
- How many times during the night do you get up to go to the bathroom?
- Do you have pain when you urinate?
- Are you reluctant to take a vacation or go for car rides because you fear that you won't find a bathroom when you need it?
- Do you avoid visiting with friends?
- Have you ever had to switch or stop your sport because you leaked urine?
- Do you lose gas or stool uncontrollably?

During your first visit to a clinician, you should also be asked about any related urinary symptoms and habits. Symptoms can be classified as obstructive or irritative. Obstructive symptoms include hesitancy (difficulty starting the stream of urine), dribbling (an involuntary loss of urine at the conclusion of voiding, which occurs in drops or in an unsteady stream), intermittency (a stopping and starting of the urinary stream due to the inability to complete voiding and empty the bladder on one single bladder contraction), and sensation of incomplete emptying. Irritative symptoms include nocturia (frequent awakenings at night to urinate), frequency, urgency, and dysuria (painful urination). Obstructive symptoms often require referral to a urologic specialist, whereas irritative symptoms can often be controlled by nonsurgical treatments.

During your medical examination there are details about your incontinence which the clinician should discuss with you. The AHCPR (Agency for Health Care Policy and Research) clinical practice guidelines we discussed in Chapter 6 contain a basic medical history evaluation chart. Read over this list so that you can take all the necessary information with you when you visit your clinician.

AHCPR BASIC
EVALUATION CHECKLIST

The AHCPR developed an outline for a clinical assessment of persons with incontinence. The following are the specifics for that assessment.

- Compilation of an incontinence profile, including the duration and characteristics of your incontinence.
- Your most bothersome symptoms.
- Frequency, timing, amount of urine leakage, incontinence episodes.

- Time of day when the incontinence occurs—during day, night, or both?
- Is there a sense of incomplete emptying?
- Is straining when voiding a problem?
- Presence of factors which precipitate incontinence—laughing, coughing, exercise, effects of surgery, recent illness, medications.
- Urinary tract symptoms such as nocturia, hesitancy, straining, pain, and so on.
- Daily fluid intake.
- Bowel habits.
- Changes in sexual habits.
- Number and type of absorbent pads used.
- Previous treatment and its effect on your UI. Especially important is any previous pelvic or back surgery.
- Your expectations of treatment.

Your history will include questions about pelvic floor relaxation. Symptoms may include bearing-down sensation, bilateral (both sides) groin pain, low back pain, difficulty and discomfort during intercourse, any protrusion from the vagina, and difficulty with stool defecation.

INVESTIGATING YOUR
MEDICAL HISTORY

Your medical history contains a record of conditions which could have a direct effect on the causes of your incontinence. Significant entries in your record include:

- For women, the number of pregnancies and births, weight of child, episiotomy, vaginal or Cesarean delivery.
- Radiation therapy to the pelvic area and cystitis.
- For men, prostate surgery, prostate enlargement.
- Recurring urinary tract infections.
- Bladder repair surgery.
- Urethral dilations.
- Previous incontinence treatment and results.
- Previous pelvic or vaginal surgery; women who undergo hysterectomy are 40 percent more likely to suffer from chronic urinary incontinence as they grow older.
- Current medications you are taking, including over-the-counter medications, laxatives, sleeping pills, and vitamins, as well as prescribed medicines.

At any age, continence depends on adequate mobility, memory, manual dexterity, and a healthy lower urinary tract. Part of your examination should include observing your ability to toilet. The ability to reach and use the toilet appropriately is a basic skill for the maintenance of continence. The time needed to reach the toilet, to undress, and to position yourself for correct voiding is measured. If you are physically handicapped, transfer skills are important. The clinician may ask you to demonstrate getting on and off the toilet.

An assessment of memory is an important part of the evaluation of the older person. If memory loss is present, the person may fail to grasp the significance of signals of urgency or the social significance of continence. There are tests called mental exams that can be performed to determine any significant memory loss. During a mental assessment, the clinician may attempt to determine if you comprehend questions and can interpret sensations. Also, the clinician will want to check if your short- and long-term memory is intact.

THE EXAMINATION IS THE KEY

To determine the existence and extent of an incontinence problem, your abdomen, pelvis, rectum, and nervous system will be carefully examined.

During a general examination, the clinician can detect conditions such as lower extremity edema (swelling in your legs and feet). Edema contributes to the increased passage of fluids through your blood while lying down or during sleep, causing increased urine production from the kidneys to flow to your bladder. Many times this increased amount of urine contributes to your incontinence. You may experience nocturia, the need to get up at night to urinate, and enuresis, incontinence during sleep. Your clinician looks for any neurologic abnormalities that may suggest multiple sclerosis, stroke, spinal cord compression, or other neurologic conditions. Neurologic conditions interrupt or weaken the nerve pathways to your bladder, causing the bladder to lose urine or not to empty completely. Assessment of a person who is frail and has difficulty walking includes a review of mobility, memory, and ability to use his or her hands as needed to toilet.

We have discussed the need for manual dexterity when self-toileting. The clinician may ask you to demonstrate fastening and unfastening your clothing, especially manipulating buttons, belts, zippers, snaps, and hooks, and also watch you pull your clothing up and down. Simple movements like reaching for toilet paper and wiping the perineum may be difficult for older adults or disabled persons who have decreased fine motor skills. The clinician may also want to observe you placing a pad or absorbent product.

An examination of your abdomen (stomach) is performed to detect the presence of bowel sounds, masses, and bladder fullness or tenderness above the pubic area. Bowel sounds may be absent in persons who have bowel problems like constipation. Bladder fullness may suggest that the bladder is not emptying completely.

For women, a pelvic examination is conducted, with the woman lying on her back with her legs raised and separated and knees bent. A complete pelvic examination allows the clinician to determine the presence of atrophic (wasting away of muscles and tissue) changes, pelvic organ prolapse (dropping or falling of pelvic organs—uterus, bladder, rectum), perineal (area between the thighs) skin condition, and any changes in the vagina, uterus, or bladder. Women who have changes in the tissue inside and outside of the vagina may complain of burning when urinating, itching, and frequent urination. These symptoms can lead to incontinence. Women with pelvic organ prolapse may complain of urinary urgency and frequency and describe a bulging feeling in their vaginas. If you have a prolapse, the clinician may also want to examine you standing with one foot on a chair or stool. In this position the prolapse may become more pronounced. The different types of pelvic organ prolapse are:

- Cystocele: The anterior wall of the vagina with the bladder above it bulges into the vagina.
- Uterine prolapse: The uterus and cervix bulges into the vagina. Often associated with a cystocele.
- Rectocele: Bulging of the posterior wall of the vagina together with the rectum behind it into the vagina.

Women with large uterine fibroids can have urinary symptoms and incontinence. In postmenopausal women, loss of color, dryness, and tenderness in the area of the vagina and urethra are indications of the decrease of the hormone estrogen. In most women organs in the pelvic area have shifted to some degree, which may not relate in any way to urinary incontinence. Childbirth, heavy lifting, chronic straining during bowel movements, and loss of estrogen contribute to pelvic prolapse. A pessary, a nonsurgical treatment, can be used as pelvic support. This device is inserted in the vagina and rests against the cervix, similar to the contraceptive diaphragm. The use of a pessary is discussed in Chapter 18.

It is important to find out the strength of the pelvic floor muscle during the pelvic exam. A weak muscle may contribute to or cause incontinence. The clinician will ask a woman to tighten her muscle during the internal examination by squeezing or pulling in and upward with her vaginal muscles in short, fast contractions called "flicks." It is important to realize that when asked to contract the pelvic muscle, many women will either use muscles other than the pelvic muscle or will bear down or push as they do during a bowel movement.

In men and women, a rectal exam is performed to assess for painful hemorrhoids, stool impaction (hard stool in the rectum), rectal sphincter tone, and sensation. Hard stools are a sign of fecal impaction and constipation problems. Rectal sphincter muscle tone and amount of sensation in the area are also determined. If a person has a weak rectal tone or decreased sensation, this can cause fecal incontinence. In men, the rectal examination is performed with the man lying on his left side with his leg bent. Women are examined lying on their backs with knees bent.

In men, a genital examination is performed to evaluate skin condition and detect abnormalities of the penis, scrotum, and perineal skin. This type of examination is important to determine if there is any skin breakdown, swelling, or enlargement of the penis and scrotum. The rectal examination should also include an assessment of the size, consistency, and contour of the prostate. A large prostate may prevent the bladder from completely emptying, with subsequent incontinence. If an abnormal or enlarged prostate is discovered, the man should be seen by a urologist. It is also important to check the pelvic muscle tone of men. A man can be taught pelvic muscle exercises at the time of the rectal examination.

CHAPTER 12

THE BLADDER DIARY

As part of determining the history and specifics of your incontinence, your doctor or nurse needs a "picture" of your problem. You can provide this picture by keeping a bladder diary or bladder record.

Most of us don't pay much attention to the number of times we urinate during a day. We've developed comfortable urinary voiding patterns, and only when we're forced to deviate from them is our awareness heightened. Special circumstances—the unavailability of a rest room, an illness, or a persistent incontinence condition—abruptly turn our attention to our bladder needs. If you

- have suddenly started having urinary accidents,
- can't determine why the accidents have begun,
- can't control your bladder or your bowels,
- think you may be incontinent for any reason,

a bladder diary is a good way to help plan a course of action for control of your problem. Keep a bladder diary for three to five days or longer. Based on the urination patterns you record, you and the clinician can consult about a plan of action.

REVIEWING YOUR DIARY
WITH THE EXPERTS

As the first step to managing incontinence, a bladder diary or bladder record pinpoints the frequency and pattern of incontinence episodes. Keeping a written diary concentrates attention on the bladder control center messages sent out by the brain to your bladder. It is a reliable demonstration of the severity of an incontinence problem. The record also gives clues both to you and the clinician as to how much UI is affecting the social and hygienic areas of your life and how it generally impacts your lifestyle.

Good Advice

Note incontinence episodes as they occur. It is best not to wait until the end of the day to jot everything down at one time. We all have some days when we can't seem to remember anything we've done.

The correlation between voiding (urination) patterns and urine leakage helps the clinician determine your baseline voiding patterns. It is an important part of your treatment.

The bladder record is easy to complete. These records will be reviewed with you each time you visit your doctor or nurse.

COMPLETING A
BLADDER RECORD

This book contains a blank bladder record for you to copy and use to keep track of your bladder patterns. Three examples of completed bladder records are also included to help give you an idea of what information you should note.

• *Column 1*—Place a check or "X" next to the time you go to the bathroom to urinate during the day or night. For example, some people get up frequently during the night to urinate. Others may go to the bathroom every time they hear running water.

• *Column 2*—Note each time you leak urine. Use the following code to indicate the amount of urine: S = Slightly damp; M = Pad or underwear definitely wet, at least a tablespoon; L = Wet outer garments, large urine loss. (If you wear pads, it may be difficult to keep track of how much you leak, whether a small amount or so much that you have to change your pad or diaper.)

• *Column 3*—Describe the activity you were doing when the accident occurred such as laughing, running, lifting a heavy object, or getting to the bathroom.

• *Column 4*—Note the type of liquid intake (coffee, water, and so on) and estimated amount (for example, 1 cup) you drank before the accident . Many people falsely believe that by drinking fewer liquids, they will cut down on incidents of urine leakage. That is a fallacy, because if you restrict what you drink you will become dehydrated. Dehydration is a real danger; when the body lacks sufficient fluids, serious health problems can develop. As we've mentioned, eight 8-ounce glasses of fluid are the recommended daily fluid intake. Avoid alcohol and drinks containing caffeine (coffee, soda, tea) because they are bladder irritants.

You should also record any important factors regarding each incident. This helps you and the clinician determine its causes.

BLADDER RECORD

Name: _____ Date _____

INSTRUCTIONS

Column 1: Place an X each time you go to the bathroom to empty your bladder, or urinate.

Column 2: Each time you leak urine, use the following code to indicate the amount of urine.
   S = Slightly damp;
   M = Pad or underwear definitely wet, at least a tablespoon;
   L = Wet outer garments, large urine loss.

Column 3: Describe the activity you were performing at the time of leakage of urine (for example, sneezing, coughing, lifting, trying to get to the toilet).

Column 4: Describe the type of liquid intake (coffee, water, and so on) and estimate the amount (for example 1 cup).

Time	Column 1 Voided (X) in Toilet	Column 2 Urine Leakage S M L	Column 3 Activity with Leakage	Column 4 Liquid Intake
6–8 A.M.				
8–10 A.M.				
10 A.M.–noon				
noon–2 P.M.				
2–4 P.M.				
4–6 P.M.				
6–8 P.M.				
8–10 P.M.				
10 P.M.–12 A.M.				
overnight				

No. pads per day _____ Type: _____

COMMENTS: _____

BLADDER RECORD—Sample Record 1

R.A. is a thirty-four-year-old woman who leaks small amounts of urine during jogging and when she coughs. Her bladder records show mostly stress incontinence accidents. She urinates every two to three hours, which may be a little too frequently. She wears five sanitary pads per day.

Time	Column 1 Voided (X) in Toilet	Column 2 Urine Leakage S M L	Column 3 Activity with Leakage	Column 4 Liquid Intake
6–8 A.M.	X X	m	jogging	glass water
8–10 A.M.				Coffee - 1 cup
10 A.M.–noon	X			
noon–2 P.M.	X			8 oz water
2–4 P.M.				coffee - 2 cups
4–6 P.M.	X			Can coke
6–8 P.M.	X	S	coughing	
8–10 P.M.	X X			8 oz. water
10 P.M.–12 A.M.				bowl soup
overnight				

No. pads per day __5__ Type: __Sanitary pads__

COMMENTS: __Pads slightly damp__

BLADDER RECORD—SAMPLE RECORD 2

M.P. is a sixty-eight-year-old woman who has diabetes, urinates only three to four times a day, and has urinary accidents between urination. Her bladder records show that her accidents are usually on the way to the bathroom. She does not appear to be getting the urge sensation in time to make it to the bathroom. She may need to toilet more frequently, possibly every three to four hours. She drinks 3 to 4 cups of coffee, juice, and water daily. She will need to cut down on her caffeine intake. She wears four to five Depends® per day.

Time	Column 1 Voided (X) in Toilet	Column 2 Urine Leakage S M L	Column 3 Activity with Leakage	Column 4 Liquid Intake
6–8 A.M.	X X	L	to BR	2 cups coffee
8–10 A.M.				1 cup juice
10 A.M.–noon		S - M		
noon–2 P.M.				1 cup coffee
2–4 P.M.	X	L	Way to BR	
4–6 P.M.		M		
6–8 P.M.				2 cups coffee
8–10 P.M.	X	L	in BR	
10 P.M.–12 A.M.				
overnight				

No. pads per day **4**   Type: **Depends**

COMMENTS: **I can't hold it**

Copyright© 1995 Access to Continence Care & Treatment, Inc

BLADDER RECORD—Sample Record 3

J.T. is a seventy-nine-year-old man who had prostate surgery five months ago. He leaks urine when he is upright, standing, and walking, but not during the night. He has stopped drinking fluids during the day because he is concerned about leaking through to his pants. His bladder records show he has mostly stress incontinence accidents, probably due to some damage to his sphincter during his prostate surgery. He wears three adult diapers per day.

Time	Column 1 Voided (X) in Toilet	Column 2 Urine Leakage S M L	Column 3 Activity with Leakage	Column 4 Liquid Intake
6–8 A.M.	X X			½ cup juice
8–10 A.M.	X	S	walking dog	
10 A.M.–noon				
noon–2 P.M.	XX	S	golfing	glass water
2–4 P.M.				
4–6 P.M.	X	M	going to car	soda-cup
6–8 P.M.	X X			sm. glass juice
8–10 P.M.		S-M	going up stairs	
10 P.M.–12 A.M.	X			
overnight				

No. pads per day __3__   Type: __Brand x diapers__

COMMENTS: _____

CHAPTER 13

INVESTIGATING YOUR BLADDER

The goal of all testing is to reproduce the symptoms that are reported by the incontinent person and to correlate these symptoms with testing. For some, these tests may be uncomfortable, invasive, and anxiety producing.

BASELINE TESTING

The AHCPR clinical practice guidelines recommend a basic evaluation for urinary incontinence. This evaluation, called baseline testing, includes urinalysis and determination of bladder emptying, which identifies bladder and urethra dysfunction. There are tests that determine bladder capacity or the ability of the bladder to fill and empty and that look at the urethra to determine its position, length, and mobility. In addition to baseline evaluation, more complex tests, called urodynamics, should be completed in certain cases. Urodynamics is simply a set of tests to measure the function of the lower urinary tract, primarily the bladder and urethra. Many professionals perform urodynamic tests using sophisticated computerized equipment. However, simple urodynamics can be performed without the use of machines. In certain care settings, for example, in-home care and nursing homes, simple urodynamic techniques provide useful information that substitutes for the data gathered from complex testing.

ANALYZING URINE

Urinalysis is a test which measures the amount of blood, sugar, protein, and bacteria in your urine. Specimens for testing are collected by urinating into a container. Blood in the urine occurs when the bladder wall and muscle become irritated, usually by an infection, stones, or a tumor. Elevated sugar may indicate diabetes. Bacteria may be a sign of infection. Frequency, urgency, dysuria, lower abdominal or pelvic pain, nocturia, pyuria (pus in the urine), urinary incontinence, and low back pain are common symptoms that suggest a possible infection. Any infection should be treated before beginning therapy. If an infection is suspected from the urinalysis, a urine culture will be sent for laboratory analysis. If the culture is positive, showing bacteria in your urine, you will be placed on antibiotics for one to two weeks. The person with hematuria (blood in the urine) must undergo further testing to rule out the possibility of bladder cancer.

PVR: WHAT'S LEFT IN YOUR
BLADDER AFTER URINATION

Postvoid residual urine volume (PVR) is the amount of urine left in your bladder after you urinate. The bladder seldom empties completely. There is usually a small amount of urine left in your bladder (see Figure 13.1). Have you

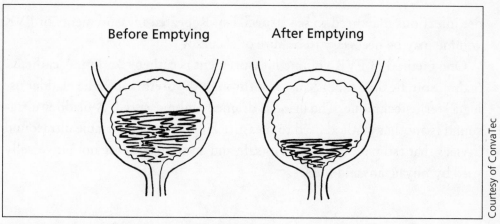

Before Emptying   After Emptying

Courtesy of ConvaTec

Figure 13.1 Postvoid residual urine volume (PVR)

ever become engrossed in a book or magazine story while on the commode? Maybe you stopped in the bathroom to urinate and find some peace and quiet. You void and get caught up in reading; before you know it twenty minutes has passed, your foot has fallen asleep, and you find yourself voiding a few more drops or ounces. That's normal! The typical range of residual urine is about 1 to 2 ounces, but in older persons it may be as high as 6 ounces.

The PVR determination should be performed to eliminate the possibility of urinary retention. Urinary retention occurs when a person is unable to empty his or her bladder completely or at all. There are two main causes of urinary retention: impaired bladder contractions and urethral obstruction. A large amount of stool in the lower colon or rectum can cause compression on the urethra, thus preventing the bladder from emptying. An enlarged prostate or a cystocele (dropped bladder) can also be the cause.

A PVR volume is done within five to ten minutes after you urinate. There is controversy about the amount of postvoid urine volume that is considered abnormal. Persons who have abnormal PVRs and who have repeated bladder infections may need to see a specialist. Repeated measurements of PVR volume may be necessary to be sure of accuracy.

One method of PVR volume measurement is catheterization. A catheter, (a thin, soft, flexible tube) is inserted through the urethra into the bladder using a sterile technique. The urine is drained and measured. A bladder ultrasound is another method used to measure PVR volume. Portable ultrasound devices that estimate PVR are very safe and accurate, but are not universally used by physicians and nurses.

PAD TESTS

The professional evaluating your incontinence problem may ask you to complete a "pad test." Pad testing is an objective way to determine or quantify your urine leakage. Pad testing is done either at home or in the professional's office. You may be given three to five pads in separate plastic bags. You take these pads home and do the following:

- Upon arising in the morning, empty your bladder and wear a pad for the next two hours.
- At the end of two hours, remove the pad, place it in the plastic bag, and seal the bag.
- Place a second pad in your underwear and remove it in two hours.
- Do the same with the remaining pads.

Pad testing can be done over a twenty-four-hour period. The pads should be returned to the clinician's office by the following day to be weighed. Another method of pad testing can be done in the professional's office at the time of observing urine loss.

OBSERVING URINE LOSS

Directly observing any urine loss is done in the doctor's office by doing a "provocative stress test." You must have a full or near-full bladder before this test is done, so you may be asked to drink several glasses of water. You are likely to void just before your appointment for fear of wetting yourself, so your doctor will stress to you that you must come with a full bladder. If this test is combined with other tests, your bladder may be filled with sterile water through a catheter. While standing on a disposable underpad with underwear off and legs comfortably apart, you will be asked to cough vigorously three times, bend, and bounce on your heels. The clinician will observe urine leakage visually or through use of a small pad under the urethral opening. If leakage occurs at the time you cough or is delayed by just a few seconds, this suggests stress incontinence. If the leakage does not occur immediately, other types of incontinence may be present.

WHEN WILL FURTHER TESTS BE DONE?

Persons requiring further evaluation and tests include those who meet the following criteria:

- Uncertain diagnosis and inability to develop a reasonable management plan.
- Other treatments have been unsuccessful.
- Hematuria (blood in the urine) without infection.
- Presence of chronic conditions, such as recurrent urinary tract infections, difficult bladder emptying, severe pelvic organ prolapse, prostate lump, and abnormal postvoid residual volume.
- Plans to undergo surgery.

After the basic evaluation, additional tests called urodynamics are performed for persons with complicated incontinence and who are in one of the above categories. Numerous specialized diagnostic tests are available, and the evaluation must be tailored to the specific problem. Urodynamic tests are designed to determine the anatomic and functional status of the urinary bladder and urethra and are performed by qualified professional specialists.

CYSTOMETROGRAM

A cystometrogram (CMG) is a urodynamic test of bladder function. It assesses bladder sensation, capacity, and compliance and determines the presence and degree of bladder contractions or instability. The test should reproduce the person's symptoms (for example, leakage of water with a full bladder, indicating a bladder contraction).

During the test you lie on your back on an examination table and have the area around your urethra and genitals cleaned. A small, soft, flexible catheter is passed through your urethra and inserted in your bladder. The procedure is not painful, but you may have some discomfort. Once the catheter is in place, water or carbon dioxide gas is instilled through the catheter at a set pace, while the machine records bladder pressure. Normally, bladder pressure rises slightly as instillation begins, then remains at a low, constant level while the bladder fills. The bladder pressure will rise steadily as the bladder reaches capacity, at which time you will get an urge to urinate. You are asked to report your first sensation of feeling or sense of bladder fullness, which is called the initial urge. A person usually has the first sensation of filling at 3 to 7 ounces of water. Then you will be asked to tell when you feel a strong urge, at 7 to 13 ounces of water. Filling to bladder capacity with a strong feeling of urinary urgency occurs at 10 to 18 ounces. When filling and recording are finished, the bladder is drained and the catheter is removed.

A simple CMG may be done at the person's bedside, if the person is in his or her home or a nursing home. This simple test is often called the "poor man's CMG" because it uses inexpensive equipment, a syringe and a bottle of sterile water. A catheter is inserted into your bladder with a large syringe attached to the end. Sterile water is poured into the syringe to fill the bladder by gravity. Again you will be asked to report your first urge sensation and sense of bladder fullness or must urge. Since there is no computerized graph, changes in bladder pressure are observed by watching the fluid level in the syringe. The water should steadily flow into the bladder. If it stops and then rises or even overflows over the syringe and the person is not straining, it indicates a rise in bladder pressure. This is sometimes seen in persons with unstable bladders or urge incontinence.

A CMG test determines the ability of the bladder to fill, store, and evacuate urine. It also evaluates the presence of urge sensation. If you have severe urgency with relatively low bladder volume (less than 10 ounces), it may suggest that you have urge incontinence. If water leaks out around the catheter, you may have an unstable (hyperactive) bladder. A multichannel or subtracted cystometrogram (CMG) measures bladder and abdominal pressure by using several catheters, two placed in your bladder and one placed in your rectum. A voiding cystourethrogram can show how muscles at the bladder neck relax during urination, and whether urethral scars or prostate obstruction contribute to bladder symptoms.

ASSESSING URINE FLOW

One of the simplest, noninvasive tests is the Uroflow (uroflowmetry), in which urine flow rate is directly observed as the person voids. (See Figure 13.2.) It is usually performed electronically, or with the use of a disposable unit. The test provides an early screening study for evaluation of your urinary flow pattern. A flow curve is considered helpful in identifying abnormal voiding patterns, especially in men who may have an enlarged prostate constricting the urethra. Ideally, you should have a full bladder when this test is performed. During this test you will urinate in a funnel container while the curve of urination is electronically recorded by a timer under the commode. This test measures how long it takes you to start to urinate, the strength and smoothness of the stream, the time it takes you to void, and how you stop voiding. Sometimes this test is done by the clinician observing your voiding. However, directly observing voiding may be difficult in persons who need to relax to void. If observed, you may become embarrassed and anxious, causing hesitancy and incomplete bladder emptying. This will decrease the accuracy of the test. If there is a delay in initiation of voiding and prolonged voiding, you may have a problem with urethral obstruction. Uroflow tends to be more helpful for men than for women.

URETHRAL PRESSURE PROFILE

Urethral pressure profilometry (UPP) measures the function of the urethra by testing the resting and dynamic pressures in the urethra and the effect of exertion on the urethral closure mechanism. However, UPP measures in the elderly may not be significant because of the normal decline of urethral pressures with age. In any case, the usefulness of UPP is debatable.

CYSTOSCOPY

Cystoscopy is a procedure that allows the doctor to look into your urethra and bladder. This test is performed in the doctor's office or as an outpatient procedure. You will be asked to urinate before the test. During the test you

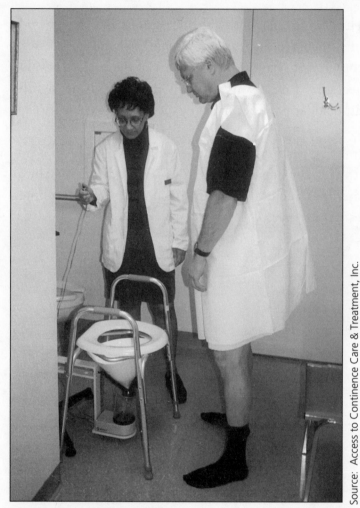

Source: Access to Continence Care & Treatment, Inc.

Figure 13.2 Uroflow testing

lie on your back and the area around your urethra and genitals is cleaned. A thin, flexible tube is inserted into the urethra and bladder and your bladder is filled with sterile water. Once the bladder starts to fill, you may feel the need to urinate. First, the urethra will be inspected for any strictures (blockage or scar tissue). Then the bladder is examined for stones, infection, or any other abnormalities. The doctor can identify bladder lesions and foreign bodies, as well as urethral diverticula (pouches or sac openings), fistula (abscesses), or strictures. Cystoscopy is not recommended as part of the basic UI evaluation, but it may be necessary for persons with blood in their urine, significant bladder infections, bladder pain, recurrent cystitis, or a possible foreign body in the bladder.

Additional studies may be performed if your incontinence problem is not fully understood by the doctor or nurse or if you have additional medical problems. These studies may include videourodynamics, which combines all of the above studies with x-rays.

CHAPTER 14

NONSURGICAL TECHNIQUES: BEHAVIOR MODIFICATION

There is not just a single solution to resolving incontinence; there are a number of possible treatments currently available. Choosing the right one is complicated, because each individual responds to a treatment differently. Treatment regimens have advantages and disadvantages, depending on a person's age, medical condition, length of incontinent condition, type of incontinence, previous treatment, and personal preferences. The attitude of the public and health care providers toward incontinence also affects treatment.

Most doctors and nurses dealing with UI start treatment with the least invasive, or nonsurgical techniques—bladder training, Kegel exercises, and biofeedback therapy. Only if these measures don't work for a patient do they move on to more complicated, invasive treatments—drugs and surgery.

YOU ARE WHAT YOU EAT

Your diet affects all of your body's functions. Too much fat leads to hardening of the arteries. Too much salt raises your blood pressure. Too much alcohol causes liver damage. Too many sweets add weight. What you eat and drink also increases or decreases your degree of incontinence.

> Emily is an emergency room nurse who works the night shift, twelve hours from 7 P.M. to 7 A.M. In order to stay alert and ready for any crisis, she needs her coffee. Emily loves coffee, the stronger the better. She also drinks several cans of Mountain Dew during her shift. The only problem she has is that when she gets home in the morning and goes to sleep, she has to get up several times to urinate. Emily wonders if the caffeine in the coffee is causing her frequency. Emily also has started to think that there may be caffeine in the Mountain Dew.

Emily is right. Persons who have problems with frequent urination and urinary incontinence are advised to decrease or eliminate alcohol, sweetener substitutes such as Nutrasweet, and caffeinated drinks and foods from their diets. Alcohol (beer, wine, hard liquor) quickly fills the bladder, causing frequent urination. Caffeinated products contain three compounds—caffeine, theophylline, and theobromine—which are part of a group of chemicals called methylxanthines. Methylxanthines are diuretics; they make you urinate. Caffeine is in cola and coffee, theophylline is usually found in tea, and theobromine is in chocolate. Seniors, especially, who drink lots of coffee and tea complain of frequent urination with subsequent urge incontinence. If you feel that your caffeine intake may be causing your bladder problems, gradually decrease your caffeine intake. When regular caffeine consumption is abruptly stopped, some people may experience symptoms such as headaches, fatigue, or drowsiness. These effects are usually temporary, lasting for only a few days. Spicy and acidic foods (Mexican food and some fruits and vegetables) can play havoc with the bladder and cause irritation. Some also find that milk and wheat products are the source of their incontinence. If you are allergic to any foods, it is wise to avoid them, too.

Here is a list of foods and liquids that might cause some urine leakage:

- alcoholic beverages, including beer and wine
- carbonated beverages
- citrus juice and fruits
- tomatoes and tomato-based products
- highly spiced foods
- artificial sweeteners

Adults should drink 60 ounces, or about eight 8-ounce cups a day. Most people who have bladder control problems reduce the amount they drink, hoping that they will urinate less often.

Good Advice

Remember, be sure to drink enough liquids.

While drinking less does decrease the amount of urine your kidneys produce, it also causes more concentrated urine. Highly concentrated (dark yellow, strong-smelling) urine is irritating to the bladder, causing more frequent urination and allowing bacteria to grow, thus causing an infection. Limiting your fluid intake will not eliminate your incontinence, but instead is likely to make you constipated, which may result in a more serious incontinence problem or illness. However, the way in which fluids are taken affects the bladder's control ability. Drinking a large volume of fluid at one time, such as at mealtime, forces the bladder to cope with the challenge of filling with a large volume in a brief period of time. This leads to overwhelming sensations of urgency. Spread your intake throughout the day, avoiding high volumes at any one time. To prevent nighttime voiding, decrease fluids after dinner.

Many of the foods you eat contain caffeine. Caffeine is a bladder irritant and will make you go to the bathroom more frequently. Caffeine is found in chocolate, soft drinks, over-the-counter medications, and as a flavoring agent in many baked goods and processed foods (although you won't find it listed on the labels). Table 14.1 lists the most common sources of caffeine.

Table 14.1 Counting caffeine

SOURCE OF CAFFEINE	TYPE	SERVING SIZE	MILLIGRAMS OF CAFFEINE
Coffee	Brewed	5 oz.	100–164
	Instant	5 oz.	50–75
	Decaffeinated	5 oz.	2–4
Tea	1-minute brew	5 oz.	20–34
	3-minute brew	5 oz.	35–46
	5-minute brew	5 oz.	39–50
	Iced tea	12 oz.	67–76
	Chocolate milk	5 oz.	2–15
	Hot chocolate	5 oz.	2–15
Soft drinks	Coca-Cola	12 oz.	46
	Diet Coke	12 oz.	46
	Tab	12 oz.	46
	Pepsi-Cola	12 oz.	38
	Diet Pepsi	12 oz.	36
	Jolt Cola	12 oz.	71
	Dr Pepper	12 oz.	40
	Mountain Dew	12 oz.	54
Chocolate desserts	Brownie (with nuts)	1¼ oz.	8
	Cake	¹⁄₁₆ of 9" cake	14
	Ice cream	⅔ cup	5
	Pudding	½ cup	6
Chocolate candy	Milk chocolate	1 oz.	1–15
	Sweet, dark chocolate	1 oz.	20
	Baking chocolate	1 oz.	25–35
Painkillers	Anacin	2 tablets	64
	Excedrin	2 tablets	130
	Vanquish	2 tablets	66
	Midol	2 tablets	64
	Darvon	1 tablet	32
Cold/allergy medications	Coryban-D	1 tablet	30
	Dristan	2 tablets	32
	Sinarest	1 tablet	30
Stimulants	No-Doz	2 tablets	200
	Vivarin	1 tablet	200
	Dexatrim	1 tablet	200

BEHAVIORAL
THERAPY

Behavioral training programs are useful in the management of urinary incontinence and related bladder problems such as urinary urgency, frequency, and nocturia. In contrast to drug and surgical therapy, behavioral treatments are noninvasive, simple, and relatively inexpensive. Many in the medical community feel these treatments should be offered as first-line therapy or in combination with other treatments. Behavioral treatments are low risk and are a particularly valuable alternative for older adults who are at greater risk for developing side effects and complications from medications and surgery.

Behavioral therapy is based upon the concept of operant learning. Urinary continence is a physiological characteristic that is learned during early childhood through a behavioral modification process known as toilet-training. We are born incontinent. An infant's bladder involuntarily empties based on stimuli and volume. An example of involuntary bladder emptying is what happens to a baby boy when the mother takes off his diaper and he "pees" up at her. The cold air stimulates his bladder to empty, and it does this despite the bladder volume. Toddlers start to develop voluntary bladder control around the age of three or four when the nerve pathways develop and the bladder control center (discussed in Chapter 2) sends messages to the pelvic floor. All of us experience these involuntary contractions during the day, resulting in a sensation of a need to urinate. Our bodies' response in most cases is to tighten the sphincter muscle, the muscle that voluntarily controls the opening and closing of the urethra. This generally results in a withholding of urination, and over a period of time, the sensation of the need to urinate passes, only to recur again at a later time with stronger bladder contractions and a greater sense of urgency. Bladder retraining attempts to teach individuals how to control or relax these urges, just as is done when toddlers are toilet-trained.

Behavioral therapy assumes that incontinent persons may have learned maladaptive patterns (bad habits) of voiding (for example, frequent urination), which may contribute to their condition and its severity. The goal of a behavioral training program is to teach the person to relearn or regain the continence learned as a young child.

Good Advice

Remember to drink the majority of your liquids before 6 P.M. as you produce more urine at night, causing you to awaken at night to urinate.

The best way to learn new behavior or to relearn old behavior is by identifying the desired behavior and gradually outlining the steps to achieve it. This outlining, or shaping is achieved through goal setting and positive reinforcement or reward. If you have ever toilet-trained a child, you know that providing rewards can help motivate the child to use the "potty." An additional component of any behavioral treatment program is the monitoring of voiding patterns and specified behavior. This is accomplished through the use of a bladder diary (discussed in Chapter 12). These diaries can be kept by yourself, a family member, or a professional caregiver. A critical part of any behavioral program is feedback from the clinician or caregiver in settings such as nursing homes or in-home care. Feedback should be provided about compliance, progress with the program, and positive reinforcement for success. There are several different behavioral treatments, including habit training, prompted voiding, bladder retraining, and pelvic muscle rehabilitation. Specific treatments depend on the individual's motivation and mental capabilities.

BLADDER BATTLES: CONTROLLING THE URGE

For incontinent persons, the urge controls them. If you are incontinent, you will probably relate to Amelia.

Amelia is sixty-one and works as an executive secretary for a partner in a large and busy law firm in Philadelphia. Amelia has noticed that for the last five years she has been visiting the ladies' room more frequently. This is a problem for Amelia because the ladies' room is on the third floor, and Amelia works on the fourth floor. Amelia usually takes the stairs because the elevator is slow and Amelia has started to feel immediate urgency to get there. But her bladder urges are happening more frequently, and Amelia is often away from her desk. She is concerned—she doesn't want her boss to start noticing that she is not available when he needs her. Also, it seems that the receptionist who covers Amelia's phone when she's away is getting annoyed. Amelia is frustrated because she doesn't seem to have a problem when she's at home, during the weekend, or when she's asleep. What can Amelia do?

In the book *Staying Dry, A Practical Guide to Bladder Control* by Burgio, Pearce, and Lucco, the authors describe the urge feeling as a wave. The urge starts as a slight sensation or pressure, then it grows, peaks, and finally subsides. (See Figure 14.1.) If you are like Amelia and most other people with urgency, you will rush to the bathroom the moment the urge comes on. You have lost your ability to make the urge go away. You can regain that control through bladder training.

Bladder training, sometimes referred to as bladder reeducation or bladder retraining, teaches you to restore a normal pattern of voiding by setting mandatory scheduled voidings that help you adopt longer time intervals between voiding. The ultimate goal of this program of behavioral therapy is to return yourself to a normal bladder function. Emphasis is placed on the importance of the brain's control over the lower urinary tract. Bladder training corrects faulty habit patterns of frequent voiding, increases bladder capacity, teaches control of strong bladder urges, and eliminates the desire for frequent voiding. A main goal of bladder training is for you to void no more than every three or four hours. To help you get to four hours, you will learn how to distract yourself by concentrating on an idea or image and by practicing relaxation techniques. You will learn how to control your urge.

There has been much research on bladder retraining in middle-aged women. It can be successful in persons with urge incontinence and those who have frequent urination. Research indicates that 75 percent of women with stress and urge incontinence who follow a bladder retraining program have at least a 50 percent reduction in the number of incontinent episodes. The research also shows that bladder retraining can lead to increased bladder volume. The bladder begins to hold more urine, and therefore you will not feel as though you need to go to the bathroom as often. It has also been shown to help individuals who have stress incontinence.

The urinary urge is a message from your bladder telling you it is time to empty your bladder. Do you have to promptly obey? No! The urinary urge is simply a signal telling you it is necessary for you to empty your bladder—not that emptying must occur immediately. The urinary urge follows a wave pattern as shown in Figure 14.1:

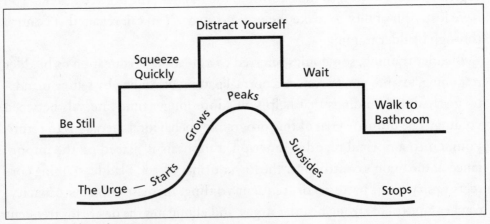

Figure 14.1 The urinary urge

Adapted from Judy Dutcher, M.S., R.N., C.S., Dorothy Baker, Ph.D., R.N., C.S., and Ronald Rozett, M.D., through Project Independence, Gaylord, CT.

The key to controlling the urinary urge is not to respond as though you've received an emergency message: "I must go now and I must go quickly."

- Rushing jiggles your bladder and increases your awareness of how full it feels, making urgency worse.
- Rushing can stimulate the bladder to contract more forcefully, making it more difficult to hold back urine leakage.
- Rushing puts extra downward pressure on the bladder, which tends to push the urine out.
- Rushing interferes with your ability to concentrate on controlling the urge.

Amelia would benefit from a six-week bladder retraining program. There are usually five components to such a program:

1. Determining voiding pattern by having the individual first keep a seven-day bladder diary.
2. Developing a fixed scheduled voiding protocol which is adjusted on a weekly basis.
3. Teaching strategies for controlling urinary urgency.
4. Self-monitoring of voiding behavior by keeping a bladder diary.
5. Positive reinforcement for achieving set goals.

Bladder retraining requires the development of a relationship between the person with the bladder problem and a professional who understands behavioral training. An entire bladder retraining program takes at least six to eight weeks before success is achieved. The voiding schedule is followed during the day; no schedule is expected to be followed during sleeping hours. The clinician must take into account your lifestyle and preferences. As Amelia's problem occurs during work hours, her bladder retraining program will target her behavior during those hours. Once a voiding schedule has been identified, you should make every effort to stick to the schedule exactly as prescribed and not to veer off schedule even if you get bladder urgency. What do you do if you get the urge to void and it's not time according to your schedule? You practice strategies for controlling urgency. You learn how to relax!

Relax, Relax

Learning to relax lessens the strong urge sensation and allows you to wait longer before using the toilet. The urge sensation is a feeling, nothing more. You will then stop the bad habit of frequent voiding, improve your ability to stop urinary incontinence, and cut down on urinary urgency.

To help you control the urge to void, concentrate on another body sensation such as slow, deep breathing.

By practicing deep breathing you will find that the urgency lessens or even disappears. Deep breathing is a distraction method to interrupt the bladder urgency message from the bladder control center in your brain. You will be more successful if you practice these relaxation techniques at home when you are near the bathroom so you do not worry about having an accident. You can also distract yourself by playing mind games—counting backwards from 100 by 7s, listing the birthdays of brothers, sisters, and other close family members, remembering all the words to a favorite song or nursery rhyme. Note how long you are able to keep the urge away.

Sue is a healthy sixty-year-old lady who is slightly overweight. She is usually up six to seven times during the night to urinate and during the day, urinates at least every hour. Sue had a terrible experience when she and her husband were at the symphony. In the middle of the first movement Sue had a very intense need to void; she excused herself and had to crawl past six persons in her row to get out to the bathroom. She voided, went back into the concert, and within fifteen minutes had another intense urge. She again excused herself and crawled past six persons to get out of her row and to the bathroom. When she returned, within thirty minutes she had to go again! This time her husband became very angry and people in her row made it even more difficult for Sue to get out. Sue was extremely embarrassed—this time when she got to the bathroom she found she had wet herself. She decided to leave and went home without her husband.

Once the urge is gone or not as strong, you should try not to void until your next scheduled time. If you get a strong urge and it is not your scheduled time, practice your deep breathing and make every effort to wait until your assigned hour. If you are concerned about have an incontinent episode, do go and void, but then go back to your schedule. If this occurs often, discuss it with your clinician; perhaps your schedule needs adjustment. You may have to schedule less time between voidings. Always try to lessen strong urge sensations before toileting. Once the urge has lessened or disappeared, then walk, unhurriedly—

How to Practice Deep Breathing

1. Sit or lie down comfortably and relax.
2. Take five deep breaths and inhale deeply and slowly through your nose.
3. Concentrate on the air moving in and out of your lungs and your chest moving in and out.
4. Place your hand on your stomach to feel it expand while you inhale.
5. Purse your lips and slowly and steadily exhale, until your lungs have completely deflated.

Repeat this exercise ten times each time you get the urge to urinate.

---

do not run—to the bathroom to void. In order to reduce the chances of awakening during the night to urinate, empty your bladder immediately before going to sleep. Do not be discouraged by setbacks. Sometimes during periods of increased stress, such as attending an important social event where a rest room is inaccessible, you may revert back to old habits. Do not despair! Just pick up your schedule again once the stress has been resolved.

How do you know if you are successful? Keep a bladder diary throughout the retraining process to monitor if you are voiding less often during the day and if you are having less incontinence. Your clinician will want you to bring these records when you return for treatment visits.

TIPS TO FOLLOW FOR
SUCCESSFUL BLADDER TRAINING

- Upon awakening in the morning, the first thing you should do is go to the toilet and empty your bladder.
- Believe you will be successful.
- Walk slowly to the bathroom—rushing, running, or any fast movement may increase the urgency and precipitate some urine leakage.
- Do not urinate before you get the urge to void.
- Use deep breathing to distract and relax your bladder when you have the urge to void more frequently than your scheduled time. For example, if you get the urge to void whenever you start to unlock your front door, stop, relax, and take three slow, deep breaths until the urge lessens or passes. Then unlock the door and walk slowly to the bathroom if you need to void.
- Do not drink liquids after 6 P.M. if you find you are waking up to urinate more than once during the night (nocturia).

AIDS TO HELP YOUR
BLADDER TRAINING PROGRAM

To help you keep to a schedule, wrist alarm watches or prominently displayed written reminders may be suggested by your clinician. A new product designed specifically for bladder retraining may be suggested (see Figure 14.2). This device automates bladder retraining drills and eliminates the need for a clock or timer. It reminds you to void with a subtle beep or vibration. You press the "Void" button when you use the toilet and the "Leak" button when you have an incontinence episode. It automatically records each voiding and incontinent episode so your clinician can determine your progress. The device is small, the size of a beeper, and can be worn at the waist or on a belt.

Amelia decided to talk with her gynecologist about her urgency problem. She had an examination and her urine was checked for possible infection. Amelia's gynecologist felt that her bladder and pelvis seemed normal and referred her to a continence specialty practice. The continence specialists taught Amelia bladder training and stressed to her that the goal was to break the pattern of immediately responding to the bladder urgency and running to the third floor. At first, Amelia was instructed to keep to a schedule only in the morning. Once she became successful, she extended her scheduled voiding times to include the afternoon. Amelia was not always successful, and the process took two months, but these specialists had such positive expectations for the outcome that Amelia couldn't and didn't let them down. Amelia was also taught pelvic muscle exercises.

Usually, bladder training is combined with pelvic muscle rehabilitation to enhance the success of behavioral training.

EXERCISING YOUR
PELVIC MUSCLES

Cathy had been experiencing urine leakage for several years. At first, it was just a nuisance, only occurring once or twice a week. But in the last couple of years it was occurring more frequently, especially every time she laughed, had a bad cough, or ran on the treadmill. Her gynecologist had told Cathy about some exercises several years ago and she tried them. Cathy felt she never did them correctly. At this point she wasn't sure what to do or if she should do anything about her problem.

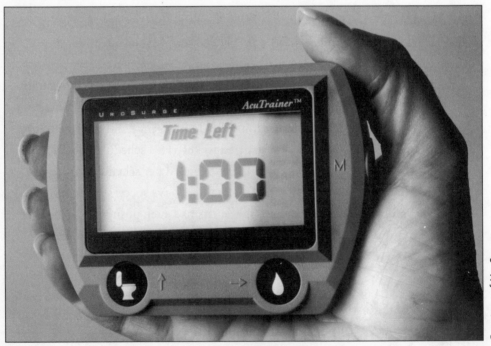

Figure 14.2 AcuTrainer system for bladder retraining

Unfortunately, for the female the normal cycles of life often bring incontinence. As we've discussed, childbirth, the aging process, and loss of estrogen at menopause cause weakening of pelvic floor muscles, damage to the bladder neck, and shifting of the uterus. Women with stress and urge incontinence need to be aware of the functions of their pelvic muscles. In men, the pelvic muscle surrounds the prostate and external sphincter. Unfortunately, after prostate surgery many men will develop incontinence because of damage to this muscle group. Urinary continence in both men and women is difficult to maintain without the strength and support of pelvic muscles.

YES! KEGEL EXERCISES DO WORK

Women and men with mild to severe stress and urge incontinence can use pelvic exercises to try to correct their problem. Many urologists now recommend that men do the exercises after prostate surgery, especially if they experience incontinence. By actively exercising the pelvic muscles, especially the pubococcygeus (PC) muscle (see Figures 14.3 and 14.4), urethral resistance and urinary control usually can be improved. These muscles act as a sling to keep the bladder and bladder neck supported, and also form the sphincter that surrounds the urethra.

The urethra is closed by the urethral sphincter and the surrounding pelvic floor muscles, mainly the PC muscle. This muscle consists of a mixture of slow- and fast-twitch muscles controlled by the pudendal nerve. Fast-twitch muscle fibers, called type II striated muscle fibers, produce strong, rapid muscle contractions. These fibers build muscle bulk. This is the type of muscle needed to produce a powerful contraction during a cough or sneeze. Fast-twitch muscles will fatigue if used for long periods of time. Total muscle relaxation must be performed between each contraction. Slow-twitch fibers are type I striated muscles that generate a less intense, sustained contraction and are useful to build muscle strength. Contracting the PC muscle supports it, lengthens and compresses the urethra, and maintains the proper angle between the bladder and urethra.

Strong pelvic floor muscles decrease the problem of frequent urination and the feeling of urgency to urinate. Repeating pelvic exercises on a regular basis increases the force and duration of bladder contractions.

Strengthening Your Pelvic Muscles

Kegel exercises (Kegel rhymes with eagle), or pelvic floor muscle exercises, were introduced around 1948 by Dr. Arnold H. Kegel, a California gynecologist. The exercises were originally designed for his elderly patients who were leaking urine. Performing the exercises resulted in such dramatic improvements in incontinence that Kegel regularly began to teach them and, as the saying goes, "the rest is history." Since Kegel originally described his exercises, they have become the first option for persons with mild to moderate stress incontinence and have also been shown to assist a person with urge incontinence. Improvement occurs in 60 to 80 percent of cases.

> **Good Advice**
>
> **R**emember, the pelvic muscles are under our voluntary control, so we can exercise them to build bulk and strength just like any other muscle group.

Pelvic muscle exercises involve training the skeletal muscles, mainly the sphincter and pelvic floor muscles. The goal of pelvic muscle training is to isolate the front part of the pelvic muscle near the urethra, the levator ani. Kegel described four levels of improvement that can be achieved with consistent pelvic muscle exercising over time:

- Awareness of the function and coordination of the PC muscle. For seniors and persons whose pelvic muscles are severely relaxed, this may take several weeks.

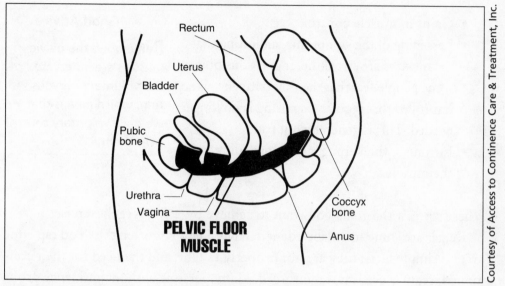

Figure 14.3 Female pelvic floor muscle (cross section)

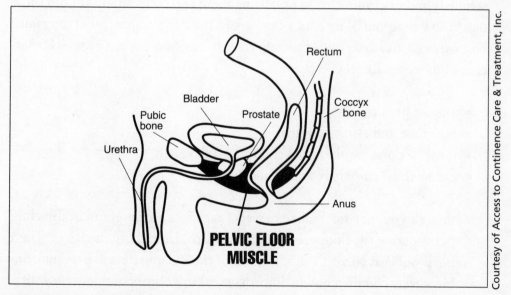

Figure 14.4 Male pelvic floor muscle (cross section)

- Gains in muscle control.
- Lessening of the symptoms, indicating that the muscles are strengthening. At this point, some people feel that their incontinence is so improved that regular exercising is no longer needed. This is generally not true.
- Firmness, thickening, and broadening of the muscles.

Good Advice

Remember, the pelvic muscles are innervated by the voluntary nervous system, which means that we have voluntary control over them.

These are just the goals you want to achieve by using Kegel exercises.

Kegels are sometimes labeled ineffective. They've gotten this "bad rap" due to two simple facts: they are not properly taught, and the need for their continued, regular use is not reinforced. Many persons with incontinence problems are like Cathy; they were taught to do Kegels but are unsure if they are doing them correctly. Anyone who tries to do these exercises has to take them seriously and be committed to practicing them regularly. Many studies show that both young and older adults can benefit from the exercises, but they must be motivated and determined to help themselves. Success can be seen 80 percent of the time. Kegel exercises:

- are not hard to do;
- take time and effort to learn;
- must be done regularly, several times a day; and
- can be done anywhere and at any time.

Although you may not realize it, Kegel exercises are taught in health clubs and spas as part of the floor exercises during aerobics and fitness classes. There is ample proof that correct and active use of the PC muscle will prevent urine loss. However, you may not see improvement in your incontinence for three to four months. Remember, it takes time to build these muscles!

BEGINNING A PERSONAL
KEGEL EXERCISE PROGRAM

Choose an experienced clinician to help you plan an individual pelvic muscle program. During a pelvic examination, you will be helped to identify your pelvic muscle by "squeezing" or tightening the muscle around the clinician's finger. This enables the clinician to estimate the strength of your pelvic floor muscles. Pictures of the pelvic floor muscles and nerves will give you a clear idea of the placement of the muscles within the pelvic region so that you know which muscle to control. Be sure detailed oral and written instructions are included in this consultation process.

Good Advice

Make sure you ask questions along the way. You should completely understand where the PC muscle is, how to do the exercises, and what results you can expect.

Depending on your needs and abilities, the clinician will schedule office visits to begin supervised pelvic exercise rehabilitation sessions. Initially, frequent sessions are needed so that the clinician is certain that you've identified, isolated, and are using the correct muscles. At first it may be difficult to isolate and flex the correct muscles, but the more exercises you do the easier it will become. You know you are using the correct muscles if your stomach, thigh, and buttock muscles remain relaxed. Most clinicians will teach you the exercises in the following way:

QUICK (FLICKS) KEGELS

Tighten and relax the pelvic muscle as rapidly as possible. Avoid bearing down or straining, holding your breath, or contracting your stomach, thighs, or buttocks.

Slow Kegels

Tighten the pelvic muscle, hold for a count of five, then relax. Direct the force of your contraction inward and upward.

Once you have the ability to contract the PC, you can do a daily Kegel exercise program in the privacy of your own home. The beauty of the exercises is that they can be done silently and discreetly (for example, while watching television). It is recommended that you do your exercises lying, standing, or sitting. One of the best positions for doing Kegels is to stand facing a countertop and lean on it. You might also investigate the purchase of audio cassettes, which talk you through an exercise session. (See Appendix A for ordering these tapes.) It's always good to have a step-by-step reminder.

You may have seen advertisements for computerized portable "trainers," claiming to be at-home Kegel exercise aids. However, their benefit is controversial and has not been proven by research. Talk with a reputable clinician before considering the purchase of these devices. There are also systems that include home biofeedback units as part of their protocol for treatment (see Figure 14.5).

Pelvic muscle support usually improves within one month after starting the exercises. Three to six months should bring significant changes. But symptoms improve slowly, and tracking symptom improvement is essential. Daily bladder records are an excellent way to mark progress and point out the success of the exercises.

How to Do Pelvic Muscle Exercises

1. *Find the pelvic muscle.* Imagine you are at a party and the rich food you have just eaten causes you to have gas or to pass "wind." The muscle that you use to hold back gas is the pelvic muscle. Some people find this muscle by try-

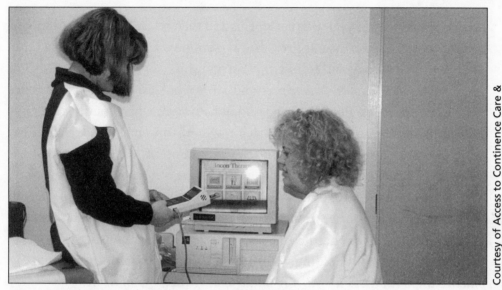

Courtesy of Access to Continence Care & Treatment, Inc.

Figure 14.5 Incon™ therapy with home biofeedback unit

ing to stop their stream of urine. Another way to find the muscle is by pulling your rectum, vagina, or urethra up inside your body.

2. *Exercise that muscle.* Begin by emptying your bladder. Then try to relax completely. Tighten your pelvic muscle and hold for a count of ten, then relax the muscle completely for a count of ten. You should feel a lifting sensation in the area of the vagina or a pulling in your rectum.

3. *If you can't hold it.* At first you may not be able to squeeze for a count of ten, so squeeze for a count of five and relax for five. In time, increase squeezing to ten seconds. If the muscle starts to tire after six or eight exercises, stop and go back to exercising later.

4. *When to exercise.* Do your exercises three times a day, ten times in the morning, ten in the afternoon, and fifteen at night. Or exercise for five minutes, three times a day. Use a kitchen timer to time yourself.

5. *Where to practice.* These exercises can be practiced anywhere and anytime. Most people like to exercise lying on their beds or sitting in a chair. Women can even do these exercises during sexual intercourse. Tighten the

pelvic muscles to grip your partner's penis and then relax. Your partner should be able to feel an increase in pressure. If you have a bladder exercise tape, listen to it twice a day and follow the instructions.

6. *Common mistakes.* Never use your stomach, legs, or buttocks muscles to do Kegel exercises. Put your hand on your stomach when you squeeze your pelvic muscle. If you feel your stomach move, then you are also using these muscles. Your legs and buttocks muscles should not move.

7. *Can I harm myself? No.* These exercises cannot harm you in any way. You should find them easy and relaxing. If you get back pain or stomach pain after you exercise, you are probably trying too hard and using your stomach muscles. If you experience headaches, then you are also tensing your chest muscles and probably holding your breath. *It is not recommended that you practice these exercises by starting and stopping the flow of urine.*

8. *When will I notice a change?* After four to six weeks of consistent daily exercise, you will begin to notice less urinary leakage; you will see an even bigger difference after three months. Make the exercises part of your daily lifestyle. Tighten the muscle when you walk, before you cough, as you stand up, and on the way to the bathroom.

If a person lacks or has weak muscle tone, there are various therapies and devices that may aid in performing pelvic muscle exercises. These can be taught by professionals such as doctors, nurses, or therapists who specialize in pelvic muscle rehabilitation.

BIOFEEDBACK THERAPY

Biofeedback therapy is learning your body's signals. For over thirty years, this therapy has helped people use the processes and functions of their bodies to improve health problems. You probably use biofeedback every day if you step on a bathroom scale to find out your weight. Biofeedback therapy is a dynamic process, really a type of information transfer. (See Figure 14.6.)

We are usually unaware of many of the processes of our bodies—heart rate, blood pressure, certain types of muscle control. Everything seems automatic. However, sometimes, all of a sudden our blood pressure soars. Our heart rates get faster. We're "stressed out" and suffer pounding headaches. We get ulcers trying to cope with daily pressures. We leak urine. Biofeedback to the rescue! Biofeedback teaches a person to see and listen to what the body says. For instance, you can use biofeedback to raise or lower your heart rate and blood pressure or reduce stress and headaches by learning relaxation techniques. In other words, you learn to listen to your body and change your habits according to what you learn.

Biofeedback therapy is also used to treat muscle dysfunction (abnormality). It teaches a person how to control the external sphincter by measuring the action of the pelvic floor muscles and immediately "feeding back" to the person information about how well the muscles are performing. Biofeedback therapy is usually performed in one of two ways: balloon measurement or electromyographic (EMG). The method you are offered depends on what equipment the health care provider has. (See Figure 14.6.) A balloon device, EMG probe, or surface electrodes on the skin are used to measure electrical signals from the sphincter and muscles. The information is stored, processed, and "fed" back to you in sound, lights, or images. Information about the status and condition of pelvic floor muscles, nerves, and bladder function is immediately accessible and can be interpreted simultaneously by both the clinician and patient. (See Figure 14.7.) The goal in using biofeedback as a treatment for urinary incontinence is to alter the responses of the detrusor and pelvic muscles, which control urine loss. Motivation and active participation play a big part in the success of biofeedback therapy.

Biofeedback therapy can be performed lying down, standing, or sitting in a chair. The position used will depend on your clinician and your progress. For incontinence, biofeedback therapy uses computer graphs or lights as a teaching tool to help you identify and learn to control the correct muscles. Biofeedback helps you locate the pelvic muscles by changing the graph or

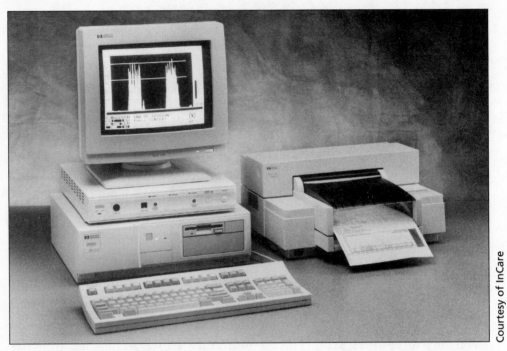

Figure 14.6 Biofeedback computer system

Courtesy of InCare

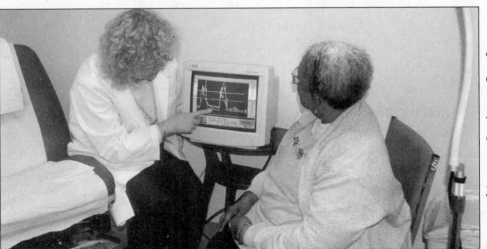

Figure 14.7 Biofeedback treatment session

Courtesy of Access to Continence Care & Treatment, Inc.

light when you squeeze or tighten the right muscle. Optimal biofeedback therapy includes visualization of both pelvic and abdominal muscle movement; thus, a two-channel system is preferable.

STRESS INCONTINENCE AND BIOFEEDBACK

Dr. Arnold Kegel, of pelvic exercises fame, developed the perineometer, a pressure-sensitive vaginal device which helps a woman identify, train, and feel successful at pelvic muscle rehabilitation. After inserting this device into your vagina, the force of Kegel exercise contractions is measured. You can then adjust your exercise pattern so that the exercises are performed correctly. You'll also learn to tighten your muscles which will help you wait to void until you get to the toilet.

The electromyogram measures activity through electrodes placed on the skin surface or sensors which are inserted into the vagina or rectum. Manometry, or pressure feedback, can only be done by inserting sensors into the vagina or rectum. By contracting your muscles against the sensor, you can identify your pelvic muscles.

URGE INCONTINENCE AND BIOFEEDBACK

During tests for urge incontinence, a catheter is inserted into your bladder. The bladder expands as it slowly fills with water. You'll be able to see when your bladder begins to contract as changes in your detrusor muscle are displayed. You then learn to relax your muscles until you reach the bathroom.

USING WEIGHTS TO STRENGTHEN
YOUR PELVIC MUSCLE

Vaginal weights (often called cones) can also be used to strengthen pelvic muscles (see Figure 14.8). They have been most successful for women with stress incontinence. They are often used as part of a structured resistive pelvic exercise program. The weights are shaped like tampons for easy insertion into the vagina and are of increasing weights. Each cone has a nylon string attached through the end to help remove it. The tapered portion is inserted first. The woman should assume a semisquatting position or stand with one foot on a

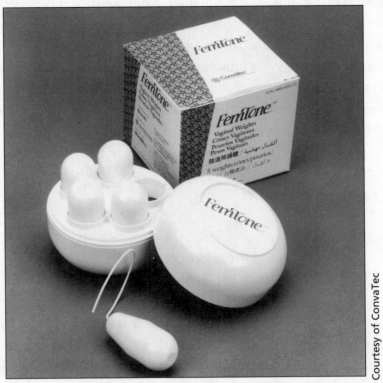

Figure 14.8 FemTone™ vaginal weights

Courtesy of ConvaTec

chair to facilitate insertion. The user is instructed to insert the lightest weight into the vagina, in the position of a tampon (see Figure 14.9). It should be inserted so that it cannot be felt protruding from the opening of the vagina. The user then walks around for up to two minutes; if the cone is retained during this time, the next heaviest cone is introduced and the procedure repeated until a cone of a certain weight slips out.

The woman exercises with the weight, holding it in by contracting the pelvic muscles for up to fifteen minutes. When she can successfully hold one cone, she switches to a heavier one. The weights are worn while standing up or walking and the exercise should be done twice a day. If a woman keeps the weight in place, she knows that she is using her pelvic muscles correctly. Holding the contraction required to keep the weight in the vagina strengthens the pelvic

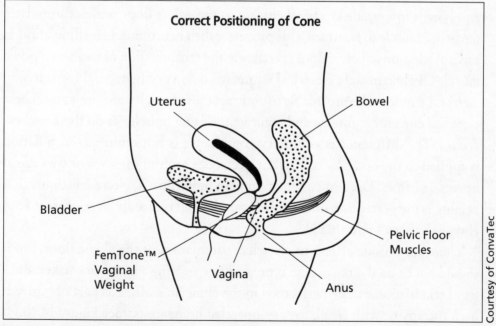

Correct Positioning of Cone

Uterus

Bowel

Bladder

FemTone™ Vaginal Weight

Vagina

Anus

Pelvic Floor Muscles

Courtesy of ConvaTec

Figure 14.9 Correct positioning of cone (weights)

muscles. To increase the exercise value of these weights, you should practice retaining the weight during coughing, jumping, or any stress-provoking act which causes incontinence.

Vaginal weights are designed for one-person use and careful washing and drying between uses will ensure cleanliness. It is advisable to wear underwear while using the weights. These weights are generally well tolerated by women of all ages. Their use is contraindicated during menstruation and vaginal infection. General pelvic floor exercises should be practiced in addition to the use of weights.

STIMULATING YOUR PELVIC MUSCLE TO CONTRACT

Applying a low-grade electrical current to the pelvic floor muscles stimulates the pelvic muscle to contract. This process, called neuromuscular stimulation, is a useful addition to pelvic floor exercises in the rehabilitation of weakened pelvic muscles. Pelvic muscle electrical stimulation is very beneficial for teaching men and women who are unable to contract these muscles on command. These electrical currents stimulate and contract the same muscles as do the Kegel exercises. The difference is voluntary compliance is not required. Stimulation is applied to the body by using skin electrodes around the anus or by vaginal or rectal sensors. Used in conjunction with biofeedback, electrical stimulation heightens the perception of the pelvic muscles and biofeedback reinforces your efforts to control your bladder.

There are no side effects to electrical stimulation of the pelvic floor, but it should not be used if the patient is pregnant or wearing a heart pacemaker. Electrical stimulation can be performed in the clinician's office as part of biofeedback therapy or with small, battery-operated home units. (See Figure 14.10.) If you have a home unit, you will be instructed to use the stimulator one or more

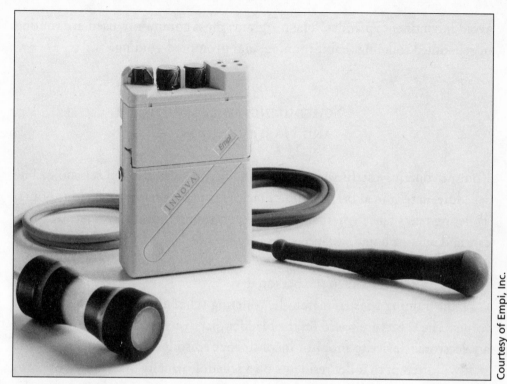

Courtesy of Empi, Inc.

Figure 14.10 Battery-operated electrical stimulation unit

times a day for several weeks to months. Electrical stimulation is usually combined with a pelvic muscle exercise program that is monitored by a clinician.

TOILETING PROGRAMS

Toileting programs are behavioral interventions that are used to avoid urinary accidents and achieve dependent continence. This means that the person with UI is dependent upon the caregiver who toilets the person regularly to avoid incontinent episodes. The programs most commonly used are routine or scheduled toileting, habit training, and prompted voiding.

Scheduling Toileting and Habit Training

Routine toileting establishes timed toileting on a rigid, fixed schedule. The schedule, determined by a bladder diary, is usually every two to four hours. Toileting takes place whether or not a sensation to void is present. In home care and nursing home situations, the caregiver will take a person to void every two to four hours. This pattern may or may not be followed during sleep hours. The goal is to keep the person dry.

Habit training tries to match the toileting schedule to a person's voiding habits. The habits are based on the bladder diary or new technology that uses an electronic device to monitor incontinence episodes. In nursing homes, the staff will attempt to toilet residents on a schedule usually determined by professional nurses. In addition, persons are encouraged to toilet independently. This type of toileting program is helpful for persons for whom a natural voiding pattern can be determined and in homebound persons living with a caregiver (usually a family member). Research has shown that for nursing home residents, a timed scheduled toileting program can be successful in decreasing the number of incontinence episodes.

Prompted Voiding

Prompted voiding is very similar to habit training and scheduled toileting except that this type of toileting program is used for persons who know if they are wet or dry. This kind of program is beneficial for persons who have few incontinent episodes, respond to caregivers if prompted (asked and taken to the toilet) to void, and can control urination until the toilet is reached. A prompted voiding program is designed to increase the person's awareness of the need to void and to ask for assistance to toilet. Like habit training, this program is for frail, ill persons who require assistance from family members and/or professional caregivers. Prompted voiding is an interactive program between the person and the caregiver, so this toileting program is directed to both. It has been used successfully for persons requiring medical care, mentally impaired persons living in their own homes, and nursing home residents. The following steps are followed by caregivers:

- A toileting schedule is developed for the person with the incontinence problem based on a review of three days of bladder records.
- The caregiver checks the person at the specified time, asking if the person is wet or dry.
- The caregiver checks the person to see if he or she gave the correct response and gives the person with the incontinence problem verbal feedback about the accuracy of the answer.
- The caregiver assists the person with toileting and prompts to void.
- The caregiver praises the person for maintaining continence and for attempting to use the toilet. The caregiver also informs the person about the next scheduled time to be checked for incontinence.

This type of program is appropriate in the in-home or nursing home setting and will be described in more detail in Chapter 20.

CHAPTER 15

MEDICAL MANAGEMENT

At the present time, the most readily available and frequently offered treatments for urinary incontinence are medications and surgery. Medication and surgery are the basic medical care for the majority of illnesses and diseases. In the field of urinary incontinence, these treatments may offer a patient improvement and even cure. However, considering the increasingly aging population, alternatives should be explored.

MEDICATIONS

Depending on the symptoms or the results of a diagnostic evaluation, urinary incontinence may be treated with medication. If incontinence is caused by contractions of the bladder muscle (detrusor hyperreflexia), anticholinergic drugs that reduce muscle contractions are prescribed. If the symptoms are the result of urethral sphincter contraction, drugs that relax the urethral sphincter are indicated. Urge incontinence and detrusor hyperreflexia are the two most common types of urinary incontinence that are successfully treated by drug therapy.

Drugs used to treat urinary incontinence affect the nerve and muscle function of the bladder (detrusor) muscle. Detrusor muscle instability (urge incontinence) may be treated with anticholinergics. These drugs cause bladder smooth muscle relaxation and increase the bladder capacity while decreasing the strength of the contraction.

The two most commonly prescribed drugs used to treat urinary incontinence are imipramine (Tofranil) and oxybutinin (Ditropan).

Imipramine, an antidepressant, has a dual action when used to treat urinary incontinence. It decreases bladder contractions through its anticholinergic effects and increases urethral resistance to outflow through the stimulation of specific receptors at the base of the bladder and in the urethra. The usual adult dose for an incontinent individual is 10 mg to 25 mg daily. It should be noted that imipramine is FDA approved for enuresis (bed-wetting) in children. Side effects include postural hypotension (low or drop in blood pressure when changing position) and heart rhythm disturbances in older persons. Persons who have heart conditions should avoid treatment with this class of drugs unless the benefits outweigh the risks.

Oxybutinin is an anticholinergic and smooth muscle relaxant. It blocks the contraction of the bladder by relaxing the bladder muscles. The recommended dosage is 2.5 mg to 5 mg three or four times a day, but dosages of 2.5 mg twice a day are commonly prescribed for the elderly. Side effects develop in a large number of individuals and include dry mouth, blurred vision, constipation, increased eye pressure, heart irregularities, and delirium. Oxybutinin cannot be used in persons with glaucoma.

Hyoscyamine sulfate (Cystospaz and Cystospaz-M)) and hycosamine (Levsin/Levsinex, Levbid, Urised) are reported to have about the same anticholinergic actions and side effects as other drugs of this classification. Flavoxate (Urispas) will decrease muscle spasm as well as having an anticholinergic effect on smooth muscle. Usual adult dosage is 100 mg to 200 mg three or four times a day.

Another commonly used agent is propantheline (Pro-Banthine), an anti-cholinergic. The usual adult dosage is 15 mg to 30 mg every four to six hours. Even in the young, the drug has a high incidence of side effects, and it must be used with caution by individuals with glaucoma, coronary artery disease, or prostatitis. Elderly clients are especially prone to confusion, agitation, and sudden drops in blood pressure (orthostatic hypotension) with propantheline. When using this medication, residual urine volumes should be monitored to avoid urinary retention.

Bethanechol (Duvoid, Myotonachol, Urecholine) is a cholinergic-stimulating drug that is used to treat bladder (detrusor) underactivity. This drug should not be used for persons with asthma, slow heart rate (bradycardia), or Parkinson's disease. Its side effects include sweating and excessive salivation, which are often intolerable. In any case, this drug is not that useful in persons with UI. Bethanechol is rarely used as it does not work well.

In persons with stress incontinence, pharmacologic therapy focuses on using agents that increase bladder outlet resistance through their actions on the bladder neck and base and urethra. Sympathomimetic (mimics the sympathetic nervous system) drugs with alpha-adrenergic agonist actions are the agents of choice. The most commonly used sympathomimetic agents are phenylpropanolamine and pseudoephedrine, which is an ingredient in Sudafed. Both these medications are over-the-counter drugs (drugs you can buy without a prescription) and are commonly used as decongestants. Phenyl-propanolamine is believed to stimulate alpha-adrenergic receptors and increase bladder outlet resistance. The usual adult dosage of phenyl-propanolamine is 25 mg to 100 mg in sustained-release pills, taken twice a day. The usual dosage of pseudoephedrine is 15 mg to 30 mg three times a day. Side effects of these drugs include rapid heart rate, elevated blood pressure, stomach cramping, nervousness, respiratory difficulty, and dizziness. They are prescribed cautiously for persons with hypertension, angina, hyperthyroidism (increased production of thyroid hormone), and diabetes.

Because of the possibility of compounded side effects, sympathomimetic drugs of one class should not be combined with other sympathomimetic drugs.

Another group of medications that has recently been given more positive attention are female hormones (estrogen). Women who have gone through menopause no longer produce estrogen. The word menopause refers to the complete or permanent stopping of menstruation and is indicated by a woman's final menstrual period. The average age of menopause is fifty-one years. Changes in hormone levels are normal and hormones can be replaced through the use of medication.

Estrogen may help women who have both stress and urge incontinence. Estrogen slowly restores the normal urethral lining and decreases bladder irritability. It also makes the bladder and urethra less sensitive, which may reduce urinary urgency, frequent urination, and urge incontinence. Estrogen restores the tissue of the lining of the urethra and thus increases resistance to urine outflow. Estrogen may be prescribed in either pill form, as a vaginal cream, or as a skin patch. The vaginal cream may have a more rapid effect on the bladder. It takes two months to see improvement and up to a year to gain full benefits.

With the use of estrogen pills, there is an increased risk of developing uterine cancer in women who have not had a hysterectomy. Most women are prescribed both estrogen and progestin (another hormone) in combination to prevent an abnormal buildup of the uterine lining, thereby lessening the risk of uterine cancer. There is also a slightly elevated risk of a stroke or blood clot. Hormones should not be used if a person has a family history of liver problems or breast or uterine cancer. Reported side effects of estrogen use include endometrial cancer, fluid retention, depression, nausea, vomiting, high blood pressure, and gallstones. Estrogen therapy can cause some vaginal bleeding, but this can be controlled by changing the dosage schedule or adjusting the dosage.

The most commonly prescribed estrogens are Premarin, Estrace, and Ogen. These pills are taken on days one to twenty-five of the month. There is an

Estraderm patch for use on a twice-a-week basis. For women who have not had hysterectomies, progestin is added during the last twelve to fourteen days of the month or daily.

Premarin is an estrogen cream that is inserted into the vagina or applied topically. Its recommended use is at bedtime, and dosage is 1 g to 4 g. Estradiol (Estrace) is given by 0.3 mg to 0.625 mg pills, taken daily. Estrace also comes in cream form. Using the vaginal cream may decrease irritable effects. In elderly women, estrogen cream can be applied vaginally. These creams are supplied in a tube with an applicator which is filled to a predetermined level and inserted into the vagina. The plunger on the end of the tube is then depressed, depositing the cream in place. One full applicator of the cream at night is prescribed for the first two to four weeks, then the dose is tapered to a lower maintenance level of a full or half applicator two or three times a week. The lowest level of estrogen that will control symptoms should be used.

To enhance early detection of any problems that may occur while using hormones, you should have a yearly Pap smear and mammogram and perform a breast self-exam at least once a month.

Table 15.1 is a quick reference for prescription medications used to control incontinence.

SURGERY AS THE SOLUTION TO YOUR INCONTINENCE

Even "minor" surgery is "major," depending on the type of procedure, your general health, the surgeon's skill, and the success rate of the surgery. There are over a hundred surgical procedures that are used to correct stress incontinence in women.

Table 15.1 Quick Reference for Prescription Medications

TYPES OF INCONTINENCE	CAUSES	DRUG GENERIC	BRAND NAME	DRUG ACTION
Stress	Urethral sphincter weakness	ephedrine pseudoephedrine phenylpropanol-amine imipramine**	Ephedrine® Sudafed® Dexatrim® Tofranil®	Tightens up bladder sphincter muscle
	Decrease in female hor-mones after menopause	estrogen* estradiol	Premarin® Estrace®	Improves condition of the urethra
Urge	Overactive bladder muscle	oxybutinin imipramine** hyoscyamine sulfate hyoscyamine	Ditropan® Tofranil® Anaspaz® Cystospaz® Levsin® Levsinex® Levbid Urised	Increases bladder capacity
		flavoxate propantheline dicyclomine	Urispas® Probanthine® Bentyl®	Decreases bladder capacity
Overflow	Underactive bladder muscle and decrease in bladder muscle tone	bethanechol clonidine	Urecholine® or Duvoid® Catapres®	Improves bladder contractions / Decreases urethral pressure
	Restricted urine flow from an enlarged prostate	dantrolene prazosin terozosin finasteride doxazosin	Dantrium® Minipres® Hytrin® Proscar® Cardura®	Relaxes bladder outlet muscle / Shrinks prostate

*May be used with urge, stress, and mixed incontinence.
**Has dual properties; decreases bladder contractions and tightens sphincter muscle.

Consider these questions:

- Have all alternative treatments you've tried so far been unsuccessful?
- Does your doctor consider your condition so serious that surgery is the best route for you to take?
- Do you lack motivation to continue a long-term course of taking medication and exercising?
- Is your condition a danger to your overall general health?
- Are you aware of the risks of the surgery?
- Do you expect a complete cure?
- Are you willing to live with any complications the surgery may bring?

It was a week before Christmas and Michelle was going to her husband's annual office Christmas party. Michelle was apprehensive as she slipped into her dark blue sequined dress. She should be looking forward to the evening of dinner and dancing, but she was worried about having one of those "accidents." Sure enough, as she started to dance with her husband's partner she felt herself leaking urine. Michelle, age forty-eight, thought, "I have on this gorgeous dress and I have urine running down my legs." A physical education teacher in the local high school, Michelle also dreaded her classes because when she jumped, ran, or shot a basket, she lost urine. She had to change her gym shorts at least twice a day unless she wore those "large"

Good Advice

Before you select surgery as a treatment, it is wise to make an informed decision. Try to find out everything you can about what the surgery entails and how it might affect you. For example, surgery improves stress incontinence, but also results in urge incontinence in some patients. Also, you may want to try behavioral therapy or even medications before having surgery.

---

pads. Michelle talked to her doctor, who felt she had stress incontinence and sent her to a urologist. Two months after she had bladder surgery, she was back to shooting hoops with her class. Michelle was cured!

Michelle's case is not unusual, as surgery has been the standard treatment for women with stress incontinence. There are several types of surgery in which a woman's bladder neck is elevated and the angle between the bladder neck and the urethra is restored. Other operations return the urethra to its normal, well-supported position and restore the closure of the urethra. These operations are performed by a urologist, urogynecologist, or gynecologist. Prior to having surgery, you should have a very thorough evaluation of your problem that includes complex urodynamic tests and cystoscopy and may even include x-rays.

Early surgery involved incisions in the vagina. The Kelly plication was the first of this type of surgery. During the Kelly procedure, access to the urethra is gained through an incision made in the wall of the vagina. The doctor tightens the tissue around the urethra to prevent urine loss during stress incontinence. Because no modification is done to the bladder neck, this surgery has a very low success rate. It is not the current surgery of choice. The Kelly plication was usually done at the time of a hysterectomy and many women were not aware the procedure was done unless they asked.

The Marshall-Marchetti-Krantz procedure involves an incision in the lower abdomen above the pubic bone and below the belly button. The bladder sits behind the pubic bone and the surgeon can easily reach it. The urethra and the bladder neck are pulled up and the tissue is stitched to the pubic bone. A problem with this surgery is that because of continual gravitational pull on the urethra, the stitches can pull away from the tissue, causing the bladder neck and urethra to fall back into an abnormal position. This is particularly true for physically active women who return to sports and exercising after surgery. Additionally, any scarring to the urethra may cause the reappearance of incontinence.

The Burch procedure is another surgery performed through the lower abdomen. The surgeon lifts the anterior (front) wall of the vagina where the urethra is located. The vaginal wall is sutured to tissue (Cooper's ligament) near the pubic bone. This is a more successful surgery because the stitches are not sutured into the bladder neck or urethra and urethral scarring is minimized.

Dr. Thomas Stamey, a urologist, started using the Stamey urethropexy around 1980. This procedure is a modification of the original Pereyra procedure, one of the first surgeries that used needle suspension. The operative approach is by an incision in the vagina and utilizes a Dacron pledget (a piece of cloth) to suspend the urethra. Since its inception, it has undergone a number of subsequent modifications and is still very popular. The advantage of this operation is shorter hospitalization and decreased postoperative complications.

A new procedure called the percutaneous bladder neck suspension is becoming popular. The term *percutaneous* means through the skin. Unlike other procedures, the percutaneous bladder neck suspension involves making only two small incisions in the lower abdomen above the pubic bone. A small anchor is placed in the pubic bone with a suture that is attached to the bladder neck, lifting the tissues upward. The incisions are closed and covered with a Band-Aid. Some surgeons think there are less complications with this procedure than with other types of surgery.

The pubo-vaginal sling is another abdominal and vaginal procedure which corrects stress incontinence in women. This surgery is reserved for women with damage to the pelvic nerves and muscles. The usual cause of this type of damage is pelvic trauma from motor vehicle accidents, or complications from more than one previous operation on the bladder and urethra to correct incontinence.

The pubo-vaginal sling uses a strip of fascia, usually taken from the thigh, to add additional support to the bladder neck and to compress the urethra. The sling is surgically secured to structures in the pelvis. Some surgeons use an artificial material such as Dacron to make the sling. Women who elect this surgery usually undergo extensive urologic testing before surgery to make certain they are good candidates for this complicated operation. It is important that the bladder work normally and that the only cause of incontinence is the damage to the pelvic nerves and muscles.

Women who have surgery can expect to have an indwelling catheter and/or suprapubic tube for several weeks after the operation, until all the inflammation and edema (swelling) subside. Even after the catheter is removed, a small number of women may need to catheterize themselves several months after surgery. One problem with this surgery is that over time it can result in the same kind of symptoms that men with enlarged prostates experience, because the sling actually obstructs the urethra.

Unfortunately, the success rate for surgery is not as high for elderly as for younger patients. Surgical procedures are not without complications. There is no long-term data available to evaluate surgical procedures past the five-year mark and it is well known that with time the failure rate increases. Surgery for recurrent incontinence is difficult and may carry a higher failure rate. The postoperative patient may also experience delayed complications from surgery including bladder instability, recurrent urinary tract infections, and erosion (pulling away) of the Dacron pledget. As with pharmacological interventions, surgery may be effective for only a select group of women and may not produce lasting continence.

What to Expect After Your Surgery

You may experience some pain and soreness after your surgery, and your stay in the hospital may be overnight to two to three days. Because of temporary swelling of the tissues in the pelvis, urethra, and bladder, your bladder may not empty well. To rest the bladder and to ensure emptying, during surgery your surgeon may insert a suprapubic catheter, a small flexible tube, in your bladder right above your pubic bone. This catheter is clamped when you go home. You will be instructed to try to void normally, then to unclamp the catheter and drain any remaining urine. Usually in about one or two weeks you will be able to empty your bladder completely, and the catheter will be removed. Some women are sent home and perform CIC (self-catheterization) until the swelling subsides. In three to four weeks you should be able to resume your normal lifestyle. You should refrain from lifting heavy objects and from sexual intercourse for at least six weeks after surgery.

ARTIFICIAL URINARY SPHINCTER

The artificial urinary sphincter (AUS) is a surgically implanted prosthesis used to restore bladder control. The AUS is recommended for people whose sphincter muscles have been damaged by treatment for urinary incontinence. This prosthesis is primarily used in men and rarely in women (see Figure 15.1).

Gene is seventy-three and has been suffering from urinary incontinence since he had his prostate removed eighteen months ago. His urologist warned him before the surgery that this might be a problem so Gene was prepared, but he hates the wetting. He is embarrassed to travel with his wife to see his grandkids because he is always looking for the bathroom, and he worries about wetting through his pants. His urologist has been helpful and feels a solution will be found for Gene's incontinence problem. First, different medications were tried, but without success. Then Gene was sent to a physical therapist, who had him work on rehabilitating his sphincter muscle. That decreased his incontinence, but he still was not dry. Gene wears at least three Depends® a day. Gene wants to be dry! Last week his urologist injected some collagen

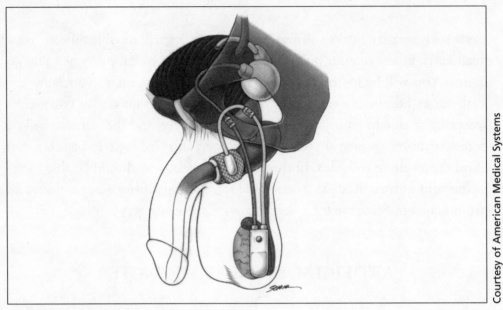

Figure 15.1 Male artificial urinary sphincter

Courtesy of American Medical Systems

around his urethra but there was no change; he's still wetting. Gene's urologist told him about a device that goes in the scrotum and penis that can stop his urine leakage. He gave him some literature and the name of another man who had the surgery. Gene is going to look into it.

The artificial urinary sphincter is a fluid-filled device that is implanted inside the body, but outside the bladder. The device consists of a cuff (collar), a balloon, and a pump, all of which are connected by tubing. The cuff is placed around the outside of the urethra. The pump is placed in the scrotal sac in males, and the balloon is placed in the lower abdomen next to the bladder.

There is fluid in the prosthesis, which is connected to the cuff through a small tube. The cuff gently squeezes the urethra shut to keep urine in the bladder. The man squeezes the pump in his scrotum to move the fluid from inside the cuff up to the balloon. The balloon holds the fluid so urine may pass from the bladder. In three to four minutes, the fluid returns from the balloon down off the cuff to close off the urethra again and stop urinary leakage. After voiding, the pressure in the prothesis returns to its normal level.

When performed by an experienced urologist, the AUS surgery is effective for a highly selective group of men with postprostatectomy UI. If you are considering this device, find a urologist with experience and ask him how many sphincters he has inserted, his success rate, and the names of other men he has treated and who have the prosthesis. This procedure is performed in the hospital as an outpatient. The cost of this procedure is around $10,000, and it is covered by most insurance plans. However, this surgery is only done with severe incontinence because of the potential for many complications.

Gene had the AUS surgery a month ago, and he feels great. It took awhile to learn how to work the device, but once he got the hang of it, he had no problem. Gene and his wife are ecstatic because Gene isn't wearing any more Depends®.

URETHRAL INJECTIONS

A relatively new treatment specifically for persons with severe stress incontinence is gaining popularity, especially for women. The body contains collagen, a protein found in the connective tissue of joints and bones that provides texture and shape to tissues under the skin. Periurethral injectables are injected around the urethra using collagen. A new medical product called Contigen®, made from collagen from cows, helps women who suffer from intrinsic sphincter deficiency or type III stress incontinence. Usually these woman have had previous surgery and continue to have incontinence. Contigen® is a collagen implant that is injected using a needle and syringe into the tissues surrounding the urethra at the area of the bladder neck. The collagen adds bulk to the urethra and sphincter to prevent urethral urine leakage. Individuals must be carefully selected for collagen treatment.

Prior to the use of collagen, you must have a thorough evaluation of your incontinence, including complex urodynamic studies. Also, a small amount of Contigen® material should be injected under the skin of your forearm to make sure you do not have an allergy to the collagen. You will be asked to watch the skin test site for four weeks to see if any redness or swelling occurs, indicating a positive allergic reaction. The major disadvantage to using collagen is the potential for multiple treatments and the very high cost of the collagen itself. The only collagen product approved for use in the urethra is Contigen®. Injections are only used in a select group and success rates are low.

As in the case of the artificial sphincter, you should only have periurethral injections performed by an experienced doctor, usually a urologist or urogynecologist.

Lee is fifty and has had a bladder control problem for fifteen years. She has sought treatment but has seen very little change in her problem. She loses urine when she changes position—stands up, sits down—and without any warning. She wears three Serenity® pads a day. Her urologist has told her she has stress incontinence. In 1983, she had bladder surgery but nothing changed. Lee has tried estrogen therapy with no results. She recently saw an incontinence nurse practitioner who works with a urologist in her hometown. The nurse performed several bladder tests on Lee and told her that she might be a good candidate for periurethral injections. Lee wasn't excited about this treatment, but she felt desperate. She could not live with her incontinence for the rest of her life. Lee had one Contigen® injection, and she was dry!

CHAPTER 16

MANAGING YOUR URINARY INCONTINENCE PROBLEM WITH CATHETERS

In many cases, surgery, medications, and behavioral treatment may not cure your problem or are not appropriate for you. You will have to learn how to manage your urinary incontinence. In order to do this, you need information about the devices and products that can contain urinary leakage. Older people and family members are often confused about various types of products, such as catheters, and their effectiveness in treating urinary incontinence. In this chapter we will review incontinence products that are available at your local pharmacy, from medical equipment dealers (DMEs), and directly from manufacturers, describe particular products and devices, discuss the problems that can arise from using them, and provide helpful tips for their use.

Medicare and other major insurers will usually pay for only a limited monthly supply of most of these products. HMOs and managed care insurers do not routinely pay for them, but some HMOs follow Medicare guidelines for payment. Absorbent products (pads, adult diapers) sold in supermarkets and drugstores are considered personal hygiene products, so their cost is not covered by insurers.

USING CATHETERS TO COLLECT THE URINE

As we have explained, your bladder is a hollow organ, like a balloon, located in your pelvis behind your pubic (pelvic) bone. It is a muscle which collects and stores urine from your kidneys and is free of germs. Some people need help to pass urine from their bladders because they suffer from medical problems that do not let the bladder empty completely. Inserting a catheter (catheterization) into the bladder is one way to manage the problem of urinary retention. A catheter is a soft, flexible, hollow tube.

A catheter is used for two common medical problems: urinary incontinence (unexpected urine leakage) and urinary retention (incomplete bladder emptying). To ease these conditions, the catheter is put into the bladder to drain the urine. It may stay in place for a short or a long time, depending on the type of catheter and the reason for its use. If the catheter is left in place for more than a few hours, a small balloon at the catheter's tip keeps it in place and the end of the catheter is attached to a bag which collects the urine. Catheters are used in several different ways:

- They are put intermittently into the bladder through the urethra (intermittent catheterization).
- They are placed in the bladder through the urethra on a permanent basis (indwelling urethral catheterization).
- They are inserted into the bladder through the stomach (suprapubic catheterization) during surgery.
- Catheters are placed around the outside of the penis for men (external condom catheters).

CATHETERIZATION ON
AN INTERMITTENT BASIS

Intermittent catheters (IC), or straight catheters, are used in persons who are unable to empty their bladders partially or completely. Causes for this problem include stroke, spinal cord injury (quadriplegics and paraplegics), diabetes, spina bifida, MS (multiple sclerosis), and obstruction of the urethra. This condition is called urinary retention (incomplete bladder emptying).

Mrs. R. is a seventy-eight-year-old healthy woman who, on a routine visit to her doctor a year ago, was found to have urinary retention. She was referred to a urologist specialist who was unable to find the reason for the retention. Mrs. R. has been on an intermittent catheterization schedule for the last six months. Because her catheterized volumes of urine average 10 to 13 ounces, she must be catheterized every six hours.

During urination the bladder contracts and the pelvic floor muscles relax to allow urine to pass through the urethra. Normally, after the bladder empties, there is a small amount of urine (less than 3 ounces) left in the bladder. What is left is known as the postvoid residual volume. If you cannot completely empty your bladder, a large residual volume builds up. This is an unhealthy situation and can cause bladder infections, urinary incontinence, and permanent damage to the bladder and kidneys. To prevent urine buildup, a catheter is inserted in the urethra to finish emptying the urine left after you urinate. The catheter drains the remaining urine, and then it is removed. By inserting the catheter several times during the day, you lessen the episodes of overdistension (overfilling) of the bladder. You usually perform this type of catheterization yourself or a caregiver or family member helps you, using sterile or clean catheters. A routine bladder emptying schedule is usually three to four times per day. Long-term use of intermittent catheterization is preferable to leaving a catheter in the bladder (indwelling urethral catheterization) because of the lower risk of infection and other problems. Difficulties that can result from intermittent catheterization include swelling of the urethra, stricture, kidney damage, and epididymitis (infection in the duct of the penis).

The nonsterile clean approach is called *clean intermittent catheterization* (CIC). The sterile technique uses a new "sterilized" catheter each time catheterization is performed. Clean technique is when you reuse the same catheter several times, washing the catheter with soap and water between uses. Since CIC is performed by yourself, usually in your home, it is not necessary to be sterile, just clean. This type of catheterization has a low risk of infection, and if one occurs, it is usually managed without causing kidney damage. Research has shown if the bladder is emptied regularly and completely before it gets overstretched, there is little chance of infection.

Older persons and those with impaired immune systems (for example, persons with AIDS or those receiving chemotherapy) are at risk for developing urinary infections, and the sterile technique is best for them. It is not known if elderly persons should also perform the catheterization using sterile catheters. The use of long-term antibiotics in people regularly using CIC is not necessary, and such long-term use is associated with the presence of resistant bacterial strains. But if an infection occurs, it should be treated. In those with an internal prosthesis (pacemaker, heart valve), the use of antibiotic therapy for bacteria in the urine is often recommended.

Anyone can put in these catheters because it is a safe and a simple procedure to learn. Older persons, family members, and/or caregivers who have the physical and mental abilities and who are motivated can be taught to perform CIC. Before using CIC, it is important to consider the age of the patient, the physical ability of the person who will perform the catheterization, and the willingness and self-discipline of both.

TYPES OF CATHETERS

There are several different types of straight catheters. A catheter for women is 5-inches in length. A catheter with a slight curve at the tip, called a coudé , may be helpful in both men and women. (See Figure 16.1.) An olive tip catheter for women may help a woman identify her urethra. Using a coudé or curved tip catheter makes it easier for men to thread the catheter past their prostates. A more rigid catheter makes insertion easier. Self-contained systems decrease chances of infection. There are also catheter guides to aid women in performing self-catheterization.

CATHETERIZATION SCHEDULE

The doctor or nurse who teaches you how to catheterize will give you a schedule to follow. As a general rule, you should drain your bladder before it has 12 to 13 ounces. You should keep records of the amount of urine you drain from your bladder during each catheterization and the amount you void. Catheterization is usually done three to four times during the day.

Before you begin, you will need the following equipment:

- Size 14 French, clear plastic, 5-inch length (for women) or 12-inch length (for men) catheter with straight or curved tip
- Water-soluble lubricant (not petroleum jelly or Vaseline)
- Soap, water, and towelettes
- Container to collect urine, such as a measuring cup
- Plastic bag to store and carry away the used catheter

Arrange your clothing so that it does not get in your way and try to urinate before the catheterization. Always wash your hands with soap and warm

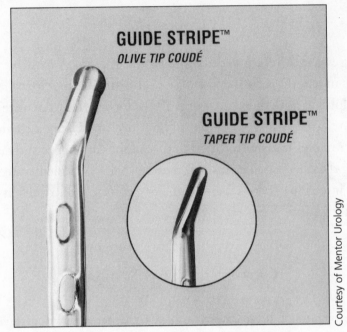

Figure 16.1 Olive tip straight Coudé catheter

water before starting the procedure. You may catheterize yourself while sitting on or standing over a toilet, sitting in a chair, or lying in bed.

CIC Procedure for Women

Instructions for clean intermittent catheterization for women are shown in Figure 16.3 and are as follows:

1. With your nondominant hand, spread your labia (vaginal lips) with your first and third fingers and identify your clitoris, urethra, vaginal

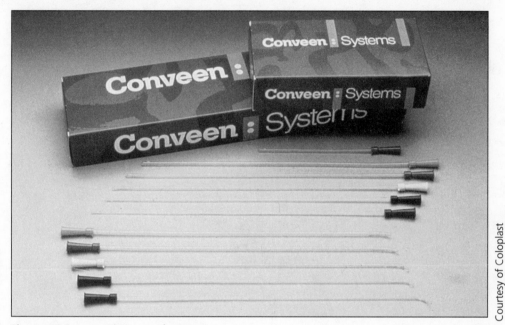

Courtesy of Coloplast

Figure 16.2 Intermittent catheters

opening, and rectum. If necessary, use a mirror to help locate these organs. Place your index finger on your clitoris and place your third and fourth finger at the opening to your vagina. Rest this hand there.

2. With your dominant hand, hold the catheter like a pencil, about 1 to 2 inches from the tip. Put it in the urethra (the opening which is located directly above the opening to your vagina and below your clitoris) until urine starts to flow through the catheter. When putting in the catheter, point it upward.

3. When the urine starts to flow, put the catheter in another inch or two. Let the urine drain. Push with your hand on your lower stomach to completely empty your bladder. Wait until urine stops draining before slowly removing the catheter.

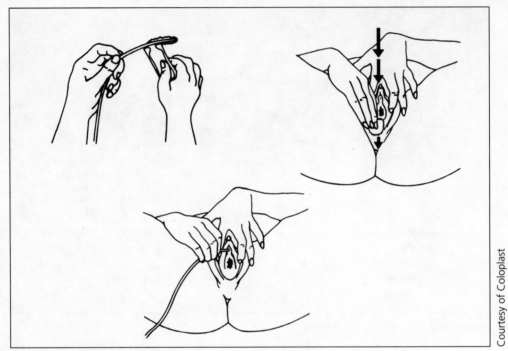

Figure 16.3 Clean intermittent catheterization demonstration for women

Courtesy of Coloplast

CIC PROCEDURE FOR MEN

Instructions for clean intermittent catheterization for men are shown in Figure 16.4 and are as follows:

1. If this is the first catheterization of the day, hold up your penis with one hand and wash the penis from the top to the bottom with soap and warm water.
2. Put a generous amount of water-soluble lubricant (such as K-Y Jelly) along the entire length of the catheter. *Do not use Vaseline.*

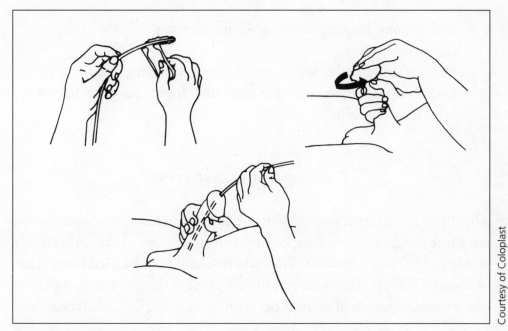

Figure 16.4 Clean intermittent catheterization demonstration for men

Courtesy of Coloplast

3. With your nondominant hand, hold your penis firmly, directly under the head, lifting the penis up straight. Holding the penis this way will make insertion of the catheter easier. If you are not circumcised, your foreskin should be pulled back and the head of your penis thoroughly cleaned.

4. With your dominant hand, hold the catheter 2 to 3 inches from the tip and put the catheter in slowly. Some resistance from the prostate may be felt halfway down. If this happens, stop and take a few deep breaths, then continue to pass the catheter gently but firmly. Do not force the catheter by pushing down on the penis. Put the catheter in 1 to 2 inches more after urine starts to flow out. Let the urine drain

until it stops. Pushing down on the bladder may help the bladder empty completely.

5. Remove the catheter slowly, allowing any remaining urine to drain out. Hold the catheter tip up as you pull it from your penis so that urine does not spill.

CARE OF YOUR CATHETER

After using the catheter, wash it with hot, soapy water and rinse with hot water. Place the catheter on a paper towel to air dry. Store the catheter in a plastic bag or clean container. The catheter should not be used longer than two weeks. If any problems occur, call your nurse or doctor or go to the emergency room, especially if you are having trouble doing the catheterization.

COMMON CONCERNS

BLEEDING AT THE TIME OF CATHETERIZATION

There may be a slight amount of bleeding when you insert the catheter because it may have irritated your urethra. Do not be alarmed; it will stop. If it becomes continuous, call your doctor or nurse.

Good Advice

Both men and women should always remember to drain the bladder with the catheter at least four times a day, about every six hours and at bedtime. Record the amount voided and the amount of urine that comes from the catheter. Do not let your bladder hold more than 13 ounces (400 cc) of urine.

INFECTION

As long as you wash your hands before catheterization and wash your perineum (area between the anus and vagina in women, and anus and base of penis in men) you should not get an infection. Catheters can be boiled between uses or washed with soap and water. Catheters should not be placed in the microwave to sterilize them. If you get repeated infections, you may need to use a sterile self-contained system (see Figure 16.5).

REPLACING CATHETERS

One catheter can be used for at least two weeks. Always replace the catheter if it becomes discolored, hard, brittle or isn't draining.

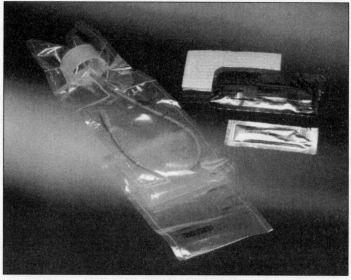

Figure 16.5 Touchless catheter kit

Courtesy of C.R. Bard

INDWELLING CATHETERS

Larry was in the hospital recovering from prostate surgery. He was going home tomorrow and his doctor told him that he would need to go home with a catheter in his bladder. The catheter would collect and drain his urine. Larry woke up from surgery with a catheter, it was uncomfortable and a nuisance. Larry told the doctor that the catheter did not collect the urine all the time. He would wake up lying in a puddle of urine that had leaked from around the catheter. Sometimes he would have intense pain in the catheter and have to call for the nurse, who told Larry the pain was from a bladder spasm and gave him a painkiller. Larry was worried about going home with the catheter because he didn't know if he and his wife would be able to manage its care.

Larry has an indwelling urethral catheter, often called a Foley catheter after Dr. Frederick Foley, who invented the device. This type of catheter is part of a sterile system that is inserted into the urethra to allow the bladder to drain the urine. Foley catheters are flexible, soft tubes that have double lumens (the space inside the tube), one lumen for urine drainage and the other for inflation and deflation of a small (about the size of a large olive) balloon. Once inflated with sterile water, the balloon keeps the catheter from falling out of the bladder. The tip of the catheter, which is inserted into the bladder, has two "eyes" to allow the urine to drain. The other end of the catheter is attached to a drainage bag that collects the urine. If you have this type of catheter, you do not need to curtail your usual activities for fear that the catheter will fall out. Indwelling catheters are usually inserted by a doctor or a nurse. The insertion of an indwelling catheter should always be performed using strict aseptic (sterile) technique, whether placed in the hospital or in your home. (See Figure 16.6.) In women it is important to clearly see the opening to the urethra, so the woman should lie on her back with her legs bent at the knees. If the catheterization is painful, a local anesthetic such as lidocaine can be used. Once the catheter is inserted, it should immediately be connected to a drainage bag. Persons who are bedridden usually prefer a bedside or overnight bag, which has a long tube. More active persons may prefer a leg bag, which can be attached to the upper thigh or lower leg with leg straps; these bags allow more freedom of movement.

CATHETER SIZES AND TYPES

The golden rule is to use the smallest catheter size that allows for adequate drainage. The purpose of the catheter is not to occlude the urethra completely, like a cork in a bottle. The folds of the urethra normally close in on them-

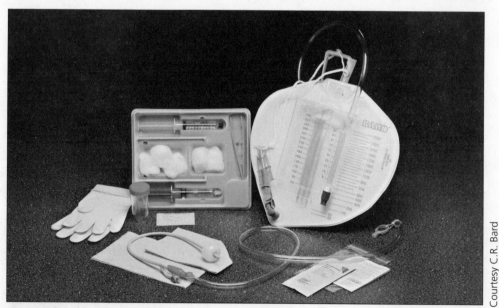

Figure 16.6 Sterile catheter system

Courtesy C.R. Bard

selves and the smaller the catheter, the more easily the urethral folds can close around it. The size of a catheter is measured in French gauge and marked as "FR." The usual catheter sizes are 14FR, 16FR, or 18FR. Size 8FR is used for children. Balloon sizes are 5 cc or 30 cc. Usually 5-cc balloons are used and they are inflated with 10 cc of sterile water. Larger catheters and balloon sizes are inserted after bladder surgery to allow for drainage of any blood clots. Most catheters have semirigid rounded tips. Variations include the curved tip or coudé tip to aid insertion past an enlarged prostate.

Several types of catheters are in use:

Silicone-coated Latex Catheters

These catheters have a latex core with a chemically bonded coating of silicone elastomer or Teflon. The coating helps prevent contact with the latex.

100 Percent Silicone Catheters

These are thin-walled catheters and have a larger diameter drainage lumen compared to coated catheters. They are compatible with the lining of the urethra and do not allow buildup of protein and mucous. Silicone catheters are now popular because people are developing allergies to latex catheters (see Figure 16.7). There seem to be fewer catheter-related problems with silicone catheters .

Hydrogel-coated Latex

Hydrogels are polymers that will absorb water to produce a slippery outside surface. These catheters are also very popular and may prevent leakage.

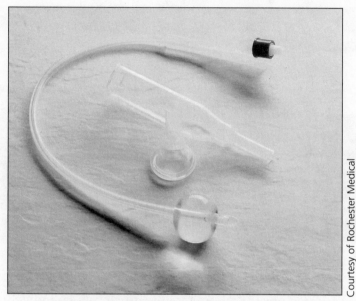

Courtesy of Rochester Medical

Figure 16.7 100% silicone Foley catheter and
self-adhering male external catheter

Previously, all catheters were a gold or white color. In the past few years, with the increased use of all-silicone catheters, they are now clear or opaque (see Figure 16.8).

INDICATIONS FOR
INDWELLING CATHETER USE

Indwelling catheters are used for persons with urinary incontinence caused by obstruction (blockage in the urethra) or urinary retention (incomplete bladder emptying) that cannot be treated with methods such as surgery, medications, or by CIC. They are also used in very sick persons when incontinence interferes with monitoring of urinary output and in terminally ill or se-

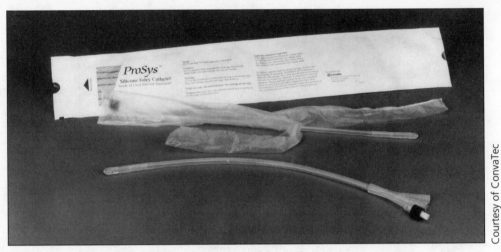

Figure 16.8 Prosys™ silicone Foley catheter

verely impaired persons for whom moving is painful. An indwelling catheter is also used in persons with skin irritation or pressure ulcers (stage 3 or 4) caused by incontinence. Catheters are also used in situations in which an incontinent person is homebound, lives alone, is incapable of self-care, and a family member or caregiver is not available to help.

Indwelling catheters are used in 2 to 7 percent of nursing home residents. Their use in persons sick and homebound is common and requires supervision by a visiting nurse and additional personal hygiene care by nurse's aides (paraprofessionals). Use by the homebound is costly and can increase medical problems.

Common Foley Catheter Problems

The most important factor in successfully managing an indwelling catheter is that the patient, family members, and staff fully understand how to monitor the entire catheter system. But even with the most knowledgeable patients, problems will occur if these catheters are used for long-term management. Difficulties can be managed if you understand the causes and solutions. Look at the case of Sol and Sophie:

Sophie has had two strokes in the past year. She wasn't able to work or move her left arm and only got out of bed once a day. Since her last stroke, she has had severe urinary incontinence. Sophie's husband took care of her, but he has a bad back and wasn't able to lift her onto a commode. The doctor felt the best solution was to put a Foley catheter in Sophie's bladder to collect the urine. Sophie has a home-care nurse visit her once a month, but the nurse has been coming several times a week for the past six months because of catheter problems. Urine was always leaking around the catheter, and sometimes the catheter fell out for no reason. A bigger catheter did not help, but created more problems for Sophie. The nurse was going to try a new special catheter.

FALLING OUT

Commonly, catheters do fall out unexpectedly. A person may pull out the catheter by mistake, or it may fall out because of too much tension on the catheter or because of bladder spasms. The balloon may still be in place when the catheter falls out. In Sophie's case the catheter probably fell out because of bladder spasms.

CATHETER LEAKAGE OR BYPASS

Leakage of urine around the catheter happens in most persons. Leakage may be due to involuntary bladder spasms (detrusor hyperreflexia), infection, a too large catheter or balloon, or bladder irritation. Bladder spasms are common after bladder or prostate surgery. If urine leakage occurs and the catheter falls out, this is probably due to involuntary bladder spasms from too large a catheter, too large a balloon (larger than 5 cc), catheter composition, or catheter blockage. Many believe that if the catheter is leaking than a larger size should be used, but this will only worsen the problem. Remember, a catheter may occasionally leak. There is no reason to be alarmed unless the catheter leaks continuously or if there is no urine in the drainage bag.

CATHETER BLOCKAGE OR OBSTRUCTION

Obstruction or blockage is the result of the formation of encrustation due to collection of bacteria (germs), crystallization of protein, or mucus plugs. Another common problem is encrustation of the catheter tip with calculous material, causing blockage of the urine flow. This encrusted material is a combination of calcium, phosphorus, magnesium, uric acid, and protein debris and occurs most frequently when the pH of the urine is alkaline. Obstruction of the catheter is the primary reason for frequent catheter changes. If blockage occurs, a person should drink more liquids or consider acidifying the urine by taking 500–1000 mg of ascorbic acid (vitamin C) per day. If your catheter does become blocked, do not disconnect the system or irrigate the catheter. If it stops draining, call your nurse or doctor.

CATHETER INFECTION

The use of indwelling catheters over months and years causes bacteriuria (bacteria in the urine) and infection. Bacteriuria develops in most persons within two to four weeks after the catheter is inserted. Bacteria may enter the bladder either by traveling up from the bag to the bladder from inside the catheter system or from the outside surface of the system. To prevent infection, always wash your hands before handling the system. To prevent infections, increase the amount of liquids you drink, including water, decaffeinated tea, coffee, sherbet, fruit

juice, popsicles, Kool Aid, lemonade, and so on. If you think you have a bladder infection, the entire catheter and system should be changed and a specimen for urine culture taken from the newly inserted catheter system. The culture will be tested to determine if an infection is present. Sophie's catheter problems may have been due to an infection.

CATHETER DISCOMFORT

Some discomfort is common with an indwelling catheter and this may have to be accepted. If the discomfort becomes too severe, an alternative should be found. If the catheter is the only option, a different type, such a silicone catheter, may be more comfortable. The discomfort could also be caused by too large a catheter mechanically pressuring or blocking the urethra. A smaller catheter will resolve this.

You may sometimes feel a burning sensation or spasms when urine passes through the catheter. This is a normal reaction and no cause for alarm. These spasms may cause some urine to leak out around the catheter. If leakage continues without stopping, call your doctor or nurse. A mild painkiller or medication to relieve the spasms may be prescribed. Spasms may also indicate that the catheter needs to be changed.

Other problems caused by indwelling catheters include tearing of the urethra, bladder stones, epididymitis (swelling of the testes), urethritis (swelling of the urethra), urethral abscess, chronic kidney inflammatory changes, fistula formation (opening between internal organs), and hematuria (blood in the urine).

Catheter Care

Care of an indwelling catheter varies. The usual practice is to change it every four to five weeks. This changing schedule is based on insurance reimbursement allowances. Persons who have problems with leakage and blockage (encrustation) might do better if their catheters were changed more often. If you think you have a bladder infection, call your doctor or nurse. The nurse may want to put in a new catheter.

When using a catheter, *notify your nurse or doctor if any of the following occurs:*

- The urine has a strong odor, becomes cloudy, or gets red. The urine coming through the catheter should be light yellow, although there may be occasional blood clots which are caused by bladder irritation.
- Signs of an infection include chills, fever above 99.4 degrees, and low back pain.
- There is urine leakage around the catheter and/or the catheter is not draining urine, which may be signs the catheter is blocked or kinked.
- There is swelling at the site where the catheter is inserted. Swelling may indicate an allergy to the catheter or an infection.

Helpful Tips for Managing Your Catheter

- Always wash your hands before and after touching the catheter or drainage bag. Wash the skin around the catheter with soap and water every day and after each bowel movement.
- Prevent kinks or loops in the catheter and tubing, which might stop the flow of urine. Do not clamp the catheter or drainage tube.

- Urine must always drain "downhill," so keep the urine drainage bag below the level of the bladder at all times. This allows the urine to drain by gravity and will prevent the urine from flowing back into the bladder.
- Anchor the catheter securely to the thigh by using an anchor strap, but do not pull the catheter tightly. Leave some slack on the catheter to prevent pressure in the bladder.
- Empty the drainage bag at least every four to eight hours or if it becomes filled before four hours. Do not touch the end of the drainage spout.
- Do not disconnect any portion of the drainage system. If the tubing does become disconnected, clean the ends with an alcohol pad and reconnect immediately. Call your nurse or doctor, because the catheter may need to be changed.
- If you have problems with leakage, spasms, or infection do not disconnect your catheter bag. However, many active persons who live at home and need a catheter like to switch to a leg bag during the day and use a large drainage bag at night.

CARING FOR YOUR CATHETER DRAINAGE BAG

Indwelling catheters are attached to overnight or leg drainage bags. A leg bag is a smaller collection bag for use at home or when you are away from home. The smaller bag is easy to hide under your clothing. Leg bags come in different sizes and are made from a variety of materials. They come in horizontal or vertical styles. The leg bag is held in place with straps, mesh, elastic straps with Velcro closures, or knitted bag holders. Be careful that your strap is not too tight, as it can restrict circulation. (See Figures 16.9 to 16.11.) An overnight or bedside bag is a larger bag with a long tube and is used while

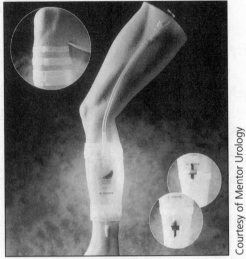

Courtesy of Mentor Urology

Figure 16.9 Freedom® leg bag

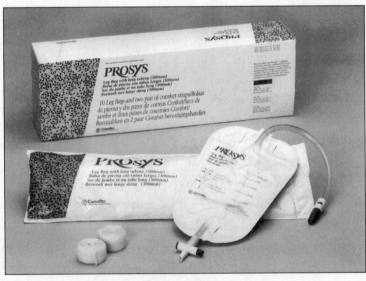

Coutesy of ConvaTec

Figure 16.10 Prosys™ leg bag

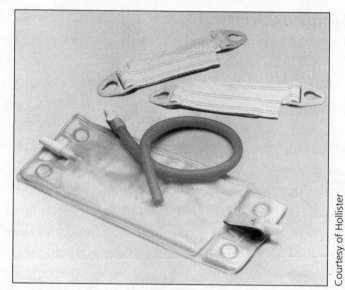

Courtesy of Hollister

Figure 16.11 Leg bag with straps

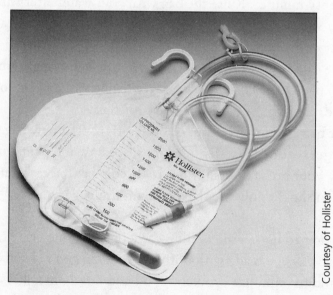

Courtesy of Hollister

Figure 16.12 Overnight or bedside bag

sleeping or during the night (see Figure 16.12). The bag should be hung over the side of the bed below the level of your catheter so that the urine will flow easily.

The care of both bags is the same. To disconnect or change your drainage bag, follow these steps:

- Pinch the catheter tubing above the drainage bag connection to stop the flow of urine.
- Using a twisting motion, disconnect the tubing and bag from the catheter.
- Take an alcohol pad and clean the end of the new tubing and the connection site of the catheter. Insert the new tubing into the catheter.
- Using an alcohol pad, clean the end of the tubing that was removed.
- Replace the protective cap and run tepid water through the leg bag. A drainage bag can be cleaned and deodorized by filling the bag with a solution of two parts vinegar and four parts water and letting it soak for twenty minutes. Rinse the bag with cold water afterwards. Let the bag dry with caps off. You can also use any commercially available cleanser or decrystallizer.
- Dry the drainage bag by hanging it with the emptying spout pointing downward. Do not hang the bag over the heat of an oven or radiator.
- When dry, recap the bag until ready for reuse.
- If your bag starts to wear out or deteriorate, get a new bag.
- If you get repeated bladder infections, spasms, and pain, you may be told by your nurse or doctor not to disconnect the catheter from the bag. You should only use the overnight drainage bag.

The decision to use an indwelling catheter must never be taken lightly and should always be made with both the benefits and risks in mind. To be successful and to minimize problems, you and family members must be involved with the care of the catheter and understand all aspects of its use. If you are in a nursing home or the hospital, professional staff must always be careful when handling the system.

SUPRAPUBIC CATHETER

A suprapubic catheter is a catheter which is inserted directly into your bladder through a small incision (cut) made in the wall of your lower abdomen just above your pubic bone and below your belly button (see Figure 16.13). A doctor inserts the catheter during a short surgical procedure. It is used for a short time after surgery on the bladder, prostate, or if a woman has a hysterectomy. A suprapubic catheter may be used in persons who need to have a catheter in place for a long period of time because it is more convenient than an indwelling urethral catheter. It may be more comfortable, less infection may occur, and has a less likely chance of falling out or leaking than an indwelling Foley catheter. It needs to be changed, just like an indwelling catheter,

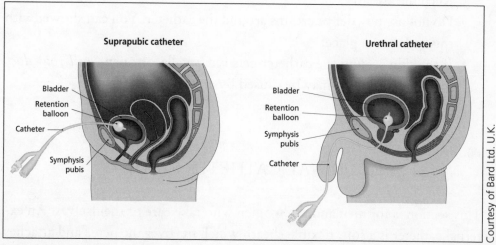

Figure 16.13 Urinary catheters (suprapubic and urethral)

Courtesy of Bard Ltd. U.K.

at least every four weeks. Problems can occur at the time of inserting the catheter, including swelling at the site of insertion, bleeding, and bowel injury. These incidents are rare.

The AHCPR panel of experts concluded that a suprapubic catheter is preferable to an indwelling catheter in persons who require chronic bladder drainage and for whom no other alternative therapy is possible, because it eliminates damage to the urethra. Management of suprapubic catheters is the same as for indwelling Foley catheters. Medical management of suprapubic catheterization may also be a problem if you are not able to find professionals who are knowledgeable about these catheters. Urologists are the specialists who know how to care for this type of catheter.

CARE OF YOUR SUPRAPUBIC CATHETER

- Wash the skin area around your catheter with soap and water every day. Keep the area dry.
- Do not use powder or creams around the catheter. You can shower with this catheter in place.
- If the skin around the catheter gets red, swells, or opens, *call your doctor or nurse*, as this may be caused by an infection.

EXTERNAL CATHETER SYSTEMS

This section is for men and the women who take care of themselves. An external catheter is a soft, flexible sheath which fits over the penis and attaches to a urine collection bag strapped to the leg. It is also referred to as a condom catheter, penile sheath, or external male catheter. These are safer to use than internal catheters because a tube is not placed into the bladder. External catheters are designed to collect urine that leaks from the penis and store it in a bag until it can be conveniently emptied. It is suitable for men suffering with moderate to severe urinary incontinence and may also be used for men with urgency or frequency in circumstances in which it would be difficult to make frequent trips to rest rooms.

Types of Condom Catheters

There are several different external condom catheters made of latex rubber, polyvinyl, or silicone. They are attached to the shaft of the penis by one of five different methods:

- Strips have adhesive on both sides and can be applied around the penile circumference (see Figure 16.14). The catheter sheath is rolled up and over the strip and penis and pressed to stick. Catheters with a band that wraps around the shaft of the penis may be too restrictive.
- Self-adhesive types of external catheters that do not require separate adhesive strips are very popular (see Figure 16.15). These are rolled over the shaft of the penis and pressed to stick. Recent new technology includes all-silicone external catheters. These catheters cause less irritation and adverse reactions than latex and are recommended for persons who have an allergy to latex. Another attractive feature is that these catheters are made of clear material, allowing you to see through them to check on skin condition.
- Spray-on or tube application of medical adhesives can give added security to the user when needed. The adhesive is applied around the circumference of the penis and allowed to dry. The condom sheath is

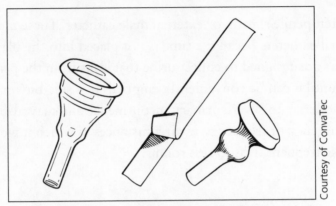

Courtesy of ConvaTec

Figure 16.14 Condom catheter with adhesive and condom catheter with separate adhesive strip

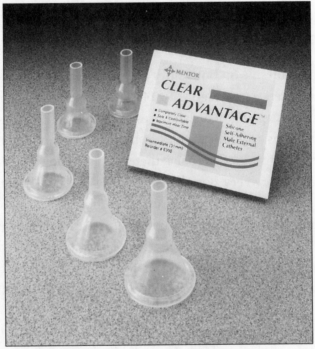

Courtesy of Mentor Urology

Figure 16.15 Clear Advantage self-adhesive external condom catheter

rolled over it and pressed down. Some men may find these adhesives irritating to the skin.

• Reusable external catheter systems are now available for the active, ambulatory man. These reusable condom catheters are great for men who experience UI after prostate surgery. The reusable system consists of a supporter brief (like underwear), pubic pressure pad, condom catheter, and leg bag with extension tubing and straps (see Figures 16.16 and 16.18). The pressure pad surrounds the penis and provides constant gentle pressure at the top of the pubic area to keep the penis projected into the condom catheter. The external condom system is nonadhesive and made of a nonlatex polymer. A tube attaches it to a urine drainage bag. These devices are helpful in men who are sensitive to adhesives.

• Some men use no method of attachment and prefer a nonadhesive con-

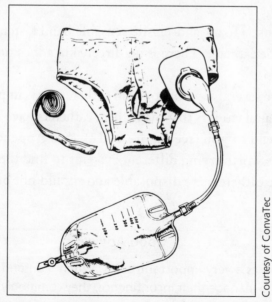

Figure 16.16 ConQuest™ reusable male continence system

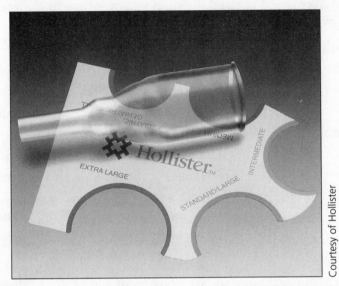

Figure 16.17 External non-latex catheter with sizing chart

dom; they use a foam-and-elastic reusable band fastened with Velcro to secure the catheter. There is no direct skin adhesion.

Since there are several sizes of condom catheters, it is important to buy the right size. All manufacturers that make these catheters have a measuring guide that they will send to you (see Figure 16.17). (See Appendix A for companies to call.) It is worth trying different systems to find the one that best fits your needs. The catheters are disposable and should not be worn for longer

Good Advice:

Mr. D.'s care makes a very important point. When men and women use products and devices to manage their incontinence, they commonly use multiple products which suit their lifestyles, jobs, and needs for security.

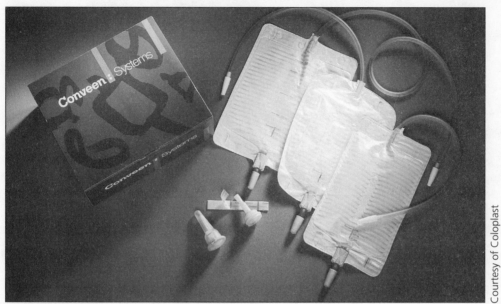

Figure 16.18 Latex external catheter system with bag

than twenty-four to forty-eight hours. In hot and humid weather, they will need to be changed more often. These catheters are popular because many men do not want to use diapers and pads.

Mr. D. recently came to my office to explore better management options for his incontinence. He had prostate cancer surgery one month ago and since his catheter was removed, he has had UI problems, especially when rising from a chair or when walking. His urologist told him that the incontinence should resolve in six months. Mr. D.'s wife bought him Depends® to wear. Mr. D. is the CEO of a bottling company and attends several meetings every day. He has severe anxiety over wetting through his Depends®. Mr. D. was given a self-adhesive, silicone-coated disposable external catheter. He returned in two weeks and asked if there was a reusable external system because he doesn't like to wear the disposable catheter for longer than six hours

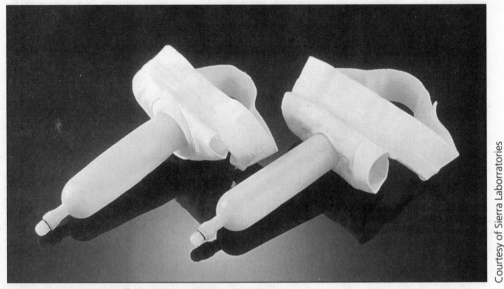

Courtesy of Sierra Laborratories

Figure 16.19 Uro-Tex® McGuire reusable system

and it pulled his pubic hairs. He was fitted with a reusable system kept in place with a combination of an underwear brief and a pressure pad. On a return visit Mr. D. explained that he now felt secure because he had three options for managing his incontinence. He wears Depends® at home, the disposable external system at his office, and the reusable system when he meets with customers.

Common Condom
Catheter Problems

Use of a condom catheter brings the chance of infection, but the risk is far less than with catheters that are placed in the bladder. Skin irritation can also occur from the friction caused by an external catheter. In older men, the penis may have retracted (decreased in size), and it may be difficult to keep a con-

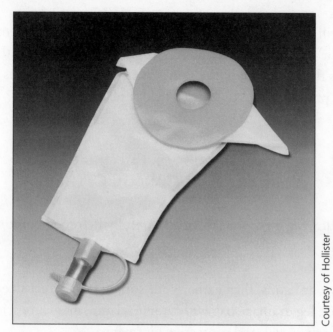

Figure 16.20 Retracted penis pouch

Courtesy of Hollister

dom catheter from falling off. There are special pouches that can be used if the penis has retracted (see Figure 16.20).

Condom catheter users must give careful attention to avoiding skin rash, maceration (softening of tissue) of the penis, ischemia (diminished blood supply), and penile obstruction. Most of these complications are the result of improper and prolonged use of these devices. Also, men who have neuropathy (decreased feeling in the nerve endings) may not feel the discomfort and pain caused by improper usage. If you are using or plan to use a condom catheter, make certain that you learn how to properly apply it and can recognize the problems that can occur with its use.

Before deciding that this type of catheter is for you, there are a few key questions that you need to answer:

- Who will place the condom catheter? Is dexterity a problem?
- Does the penis shaft have enough length to support the catheter?
- What is the condition of the skin? Does protection, such as a skin protection product, need to be used before placing the device?

Procedures for Putting on Your External Condom Catheter

Read the following directions through carefully before attempting to put on the condom.

1. Wash your hands, then gather your supplies: a correct size condom catheter, leg drainage bag with tubing, clamp, manicure scissors, soap, washcloth, towel, and protective ointment.
2. Trim or clip the hairs on the shaft and base of your penis and any pubic hairs that might get caught so they won't stick to the adhesive tape.
3. Wash, rinse, and dry your penis. To protect your skin from urine, you may want to coat your penis with a protective skin product or a polymer skin sealant and let the ointment dry (it will feel sticky). The purpose of this skin protectant is to shield your skin from perspiration and urine moisture so your skin will not tear when you remove the catheter.
4. Hold your penis and place the catheter sheath on the end of it, leaving about half an inch of space between the tip of your penis and the connector tip, so your penis does not rub against the end of the catheter. If you are not circumcised, leave your foreskin in place. Swelling of your foreskin may result if the skin is not kept over the head of the penis.
5. Unroll the catheter smoothly over your penis while gently stretching

it. When the condom is unrolled, gently press it against your penis so that it sticks.

6. Put pressure on your penis when the condom is completely unrolled by gripping it for ten minutes to be sure any wrinkles in the condom are sealed together and to eliminate any air bubbles. If there are a lot of wrinkles, the condom is probably too large; try the next smaller size.

7. If you are using a leg bag you will need an extension tube to connect the end of the condom to the bag. Ask your supplier for the extension tube. Connect one end of the tubing to the catheter connector tip and the other end to the drainage bag. Strap the drainage bag to your thigh or ankle, depending on your activities and your clothing (shorts or pants). The tubing can be cut to any length.

8. Remove the drainage bag by squeezing the drainage tube closed. Release the leg straps and disconnect the extension tubing at the top of the bag. Remove the condom catheter and the tape by rolling them forward.

CONDOM CATHETER PROBLEMS

- If the catheter doesn't stick to your skin, make sure that your penis and the protective ointment are completely dry.
- If the catheter pulls away from your skin, you may need to apply more ointment. Also, make sure the catheter is snug, but not tight.
- If urine leaks when you're wearing the catheter, squeeze the sheath to get a better seal.
- If the catheter sheath wrinkles in contact with the tape, the sheath may be too large. If so, select a smaller size sheath. Remember to allow for nocturnal erections in the sizing of the device by selecting a larger size.

- If you put on a condom catheter with an adhesive strip, do not overlap the strip when wrapping it around the penis. This may cause pressure and skin breakdown.
- Empty the drainage bag every three to four hours. Never let it fill completely to the top.
- Wash the drainage bag with soap and water. Rinse it with a solution of one part vinegar and seven parts water. Don't use the same drainage bag longer than one month.
- Do not use a leg bag which is too large, since this puts too much weight on the condom catheter and can cause the catheter to fall off.
- Use only ointments and adhesives prescribed by your doctor. Don't wash with Betadine; this can irritate your skin.
- Remember to change the condom catheter every twenty-four to forty-eight hours. Make sure to thoroughly wash and dry the penis between changes.
- Check your penis every two hours for swelling or unusual color. If it feels painful or doesn't look normal, take off the condom catheter and call your doctor.
- Call your nurse or doctor if you feel pain or burning when you urinate, have the urge to urinate frequently, smell an unpleasant odor from your urine, or see blood or pus in your urine.

External Devices for Women

There are external collection devices for women, but none have proven to be totally useful for woman in wheelchairs or who are bedridden. These devices are flexible or plastic pouches which are attached to the skin by adhesive or straps. (See Figure 16.21.) The ideal device for women would be easy and quick to place and work well for persons who transfer from beds to chairs and who are in wheelchairs. Unfortunately, an ideal device does not exist at present.

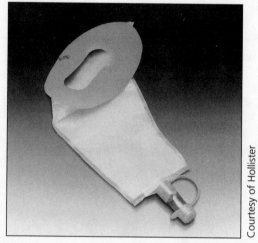

Courtesy of Hollister

Figure 16.21 External urinary pouch for women

Chapter 17

INCONTINENCE PRODUCTS

Absorbent incontinence products are used to absorb and contain urine. They include absorbent pads and garments, either disposable or reusable, which absorb and contain urine. There are several types of products including pads, shields, guards, undergarments, briefs, and underpads. Absorbent products can be a useful and rational way to manage incontinence. Many people with urinary incontinence use these products because of the protection they provide and to prevent themselves from the embarrassment from urine leakage. Others use pads because they have been dismissed rather than treated when seeking help for incontinence from doctors and nurses.

ABSORBENT PRODUCTS

Absorbent products have been developed specifically to collect urine instead of the pads developed for menstruation. They protect clothing, furniture, and bedding and allow individuals to maintain their self-esteem and physical comfort. The products are available in all levels of absorbency, from thin panty liners, sanitary pads, adult diapers, or briefs to bed and furniture protection products like bed pads. (See Figures 17.1 to 17.11.) Perineal pads are attached to the underwear or panties with an adhesive strip. Undergarments have elasticized legs with a belt attached with buttons or Velcro. Briefs or diaperlike products have elasticized legs and self-adhesive tabs that secure the brief. Incontinence products have different designs and absorbencies. They are classified for light, moderate, or heavy urine leakage and are available for men, women, or both. As there are many brands, they are difficult to compare. It is estimated that as many as 30 percent of all feminine hygiene pads (sanitary pads) are purchased for slight urinary incontinence problems, especially by young women who have mild incontinence or stress incontinence. For men, socklike drip-

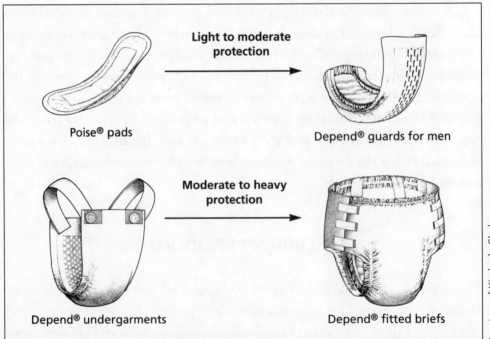

Light to moderate protection

Poise® pads → Depend® guards for men

Moderate to heavy protection

Depend® undergarments → Depend® fitted briefs

Courtesy of Kimberly-Clark

Figure 17.1 Products for the level of incontinence. Depend® and Poise® product forms are available in varying absorbencies.

Table 17.1

PRODUCTS	ABSORPTIONS (per incontinent episode)
Pad	Light urine loss up to ¾ cup, 4 to 6 ounces
Guard	Moderate urine loss up to 1¾ cups, 10 ounces
Undergarments	Moderate to heavy urine loss up to 2½ cups, 17 ounces
Briefs	Heavy urine loss up to 2½ cups, 17 ounces or more

collecting pouches and guards are available that are comfortable and discreet. These pouches and guards are held in place inside regular underwear, preferably briefs, with an adhesive strip. They offer more freedom for men with moderate urinary incontinence or for postprostatectomy patients.

Unfortunately, some of the products designed to help prevent leakage often reinforce persistent feelings of loss of independence and self-respect. Although diaperlike products may be necessary for people who are chronically ill or bedridden, their bulky, childlike design is understandably perceived by many active adults as undignified and juvenile. "Diapers are for babies, not me, and I don't like being treated like a baby," is a refrain heard from many incontinence patients over the years. Recently, an increasing number of products have been designed to fit the body comfortably and be undetectable under clothing. These disposable pads can be attached to specifically designed adult undergarments, allowing the person wearing them to feel dignified.

DISPOSABLES

Typically, disposable incontinence products are more expensive than washable products, although costs associated with reusable products include laundry and replacement. It is estimated that use of absorbent products costs

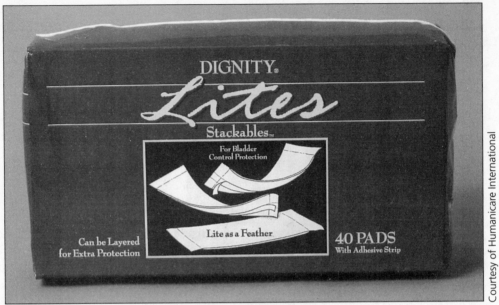

Figure 17.2 Dignity Lites "stackables" pads

Courtesy of Humanicare International

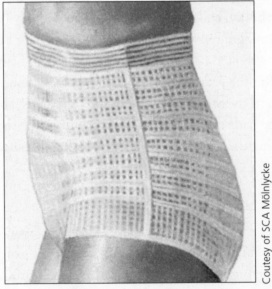

Figure 17.3 Promise® mesh pad pant

Coutesy of SCA Mölnlycke

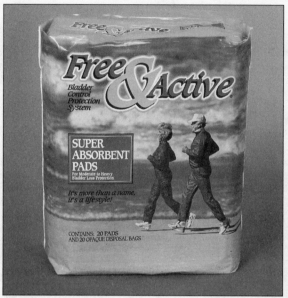

Courtesy of Humanicare International

Figure 17.4 Free and Active super absorbent pads

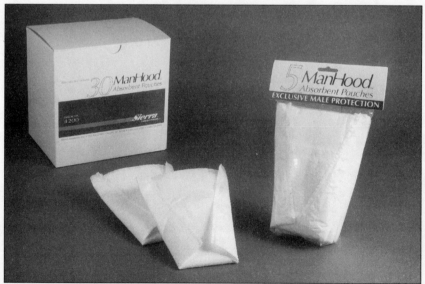

Courtesy of Sierra Laboratories

Figure 17.5 ManHood drip collector for men

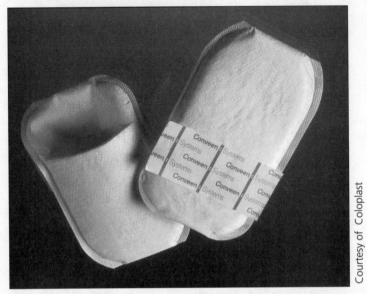

Figure 17.6 Conveen drip collector for men

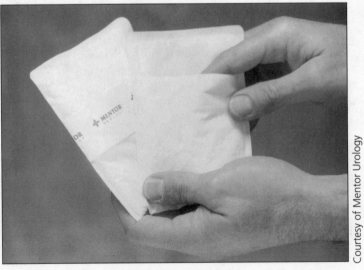

Figure 17.7 Drip collector

between $40 and $150 a month, depending on the type of product. For a person on a fixed or retirement income, this expense adds a burden to an already limited budget. Cost also forces many people to make their own absorbent pads from tissue paper, towels, washcloths, and so on. Additionally, absorbent products are not covered by Medicare, HMOs, or insurance companies, and disposal of absorbent products adds to environmental pollution.

REUSABLE PRODUCTS

Washable garments have a protective outer layer of plastic, rubber, or synthetic material. They can be pulled on, side-snapped, or opened in the front. Reusable garments are typically less expensive than disposable products. Many women find cotton underwear to be the most comfortable. Many times a perineal pad (a pad placed between the legs to catch any urine leakage) can be placed in the cotton underwear.

Absorbent products are also helpful during treatment of UI. However, early dependency on absorbent pads may be a deterrent to continence, giving the wearer a false sense of security and lead to acceptance of the condition. Their use may remove the motivation to seek evaluation and treatment for UI. In addition, improper use of absorbent products contributes to skin breakdown and infection. To avoid these problems, diapers and pads should be changed frequently to limit a person's exposure to the wet garment and to eliminate buildup of odor.

UNDERPADS/BEDPADS

The key to surviving bed-wetting is to use special underpads or drawsheets to keep the bed from getting wet in the first place. Disposable and washable

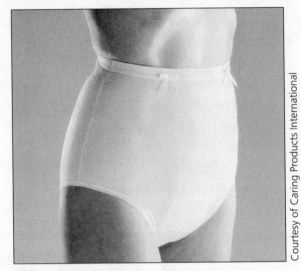

Figure 17.8 Rejoice liners for women

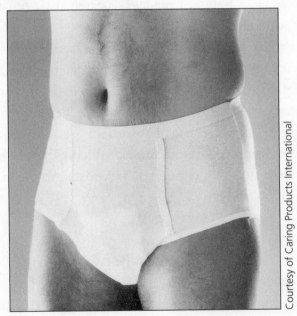

Figure17.9 Rejoice liners for men

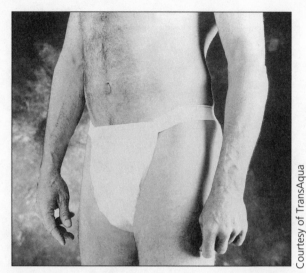

Courtesy of TransAqua

Figure 17.10 HealthDri™ washable incontinence garment

pads are available in supermarkets, pharmacies, and through mail-order catalogs. J.C. Penney and Sears carry their own brands.

Frequently patients or family members ask what the best product is to
use for protection. This is difficult to answer because there are many factors
to consider when using absorbent products. Considerations include the type
and severity of UI, personal preference, quality and cost of the product, availability of a caregiver to remove the product, and the condition of the person's
skin and its risk for breakdown. The weight of an adult and the resulting pressure on a product causes fluid that is not quickly absorbed by the product to
rush to the side, creating leaks (side seepage). Therefore, sitting becomes a
concern; women will favor one side when sitting to help avoid side seepage.

The urine-holding capacity of all absorbent products is not standardized
and varies from product to product. The quality and materials used in these
products vary widely and there is little research comparing them. At the
present time, product selection is made by the consumer through trial and er-

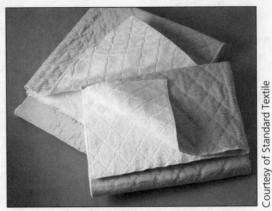

Courtesy of Standard Textile

Figure 17.11 ComPly® washable bedpad

ror, and depends on budgetary restraints and availability. Most products utilize a superabsorbent polymer that turns the urine into a gel, eliminating the possibility of leakage or odor. New techniques have produced better products that wick or pull urine away to keep the skin dry and free from irritation. Absorbent products do assist with incontinence management, but prolonged skin occlusion traps moisture, contributing to skin breakdown. Technological advances may have a significant impact on skin problems. You, the buyer, should understand that not all products have this new technology.

OTHER PRODUCTS AND DEVICES

Joe made an appointment to see the continence nurse practitioner at his urologist's office. He has had a "dribbling" incontinence problem since he had prostate surgery three years ago. It happens throughout the day and is a nuisance. A friend had told him about a clamp that prevented urine dribbling. Joe could only get it with a doctor's prescription, so he made a visit to his doctor to get one.

Joe wanted an incontinence clamp (penile clamp), a device used by men with incontinence. An incontinence clamp is placed around the penis to prevent urine leakage. Often men use these clamps after prostate surgery to stop continuous urine leakage. The clamp is placed halfway down the shaft of the penis and then tightened to compress the urethra. Skin breakdown, swelling, and strictures (scarring) can occur inside the urethra if a clamp is left in place too long.

There are several kinds of clamps . The Cunningham clamp is the one most often used (see Figure 17.12). The inside of the clamp has a flexible, soft part

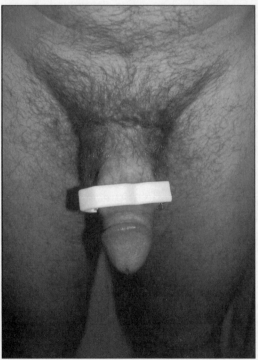

Figure 17.12 Cunningham clamp

Courtesy of Access to Continece Care & Treatment, Inc.

made of soft foam that conforms to fit the penis. The outside is made of metal with several notches on the side to adjust the tightness. Men who are in wheelchairs may place a clamp over the penis when they move from bed to chair and vice versa. They keep the clamp on and only compress the clamp when they move from position to position.

The incontinence nurse practitioner spoke with the urologist about Joe's request, measured Joe's penis for size, and emphasized that Joe should return to the office in one week so she could assess his penis for any skin breakdown. She gave him instructions about using the clamp. The nurse practitioner stressed to Joe that he must release the clamp every two hours to urinate. When Joe returned in two weeks, he was very pleased with the clamp because it had stopped his dribbling. The clamp made a small indentation in the shaft of Joe's penis, but there were no skin problems or discomfort.

The practitioner also gave Joe the following instructions:

1. Open the clamp and place it around the penis about halfway down the shaft. The clamp flexes to fit comfortably over your penis. Squeeze the clamp shut, making sure it is not too tight. The clamp must be released every two hours to urinate.
2. Look at your penis from time to time and stop using the clamp if the skin is torn or has openings on it or if the skin is pale or blue. Apply a skin cream to the penis for protection before putting on the clamp.
3. Report any discharge (drainage) from the penis, itching, foul urine odor, pain, or inability to urinate or empty the bladder immediately to the doctor, or you should go to an emergency room.

KEEPING YOUR
SKIN HEALTHY

Skin problems associated with incontinence can range from irritations to pressure sores, commonly called bedsores (breakdown or opening of the skin). Potential sources of excessive moisture on the skin include:

- urinary incontinence
- fecal incontinence
- frequent washing
- nonabsorbent and/or poorly ventilated padding on the skin

Because men and women with urinary incontinence are often at risk for skin rashes and skin breakdown, good skin care is very important. (See Figures 17.13 to 17.16.) If you are concerned about your skin and the damage that can happen from your incontinence or if you are caring for someone with incontinence, here are some basic steps to follow:

- Look at the skin carefully every day; separate any skin folds or wrinkles and look for rash, irritation, or skin breakdown.
- Wash the skin with a mild soap (such as Dove) or perineal wash product that will not harm it. Always wash the skin after any urine or bowel incontinence episode.

Good Advice

Caution! If you use a penile clamp, it must be taken off at least every three hours so that you can urinate. If you don't do this, the bladder becomes full (overdistended), and you may develop bladder problems and severe infections.

- After washing, let the skin dry rather than rubbing with a towel to avoid irritation and skin tears.
- Use moisturizers to replace moisture to skin and topical skin products that protect the skin from moisture (skin barrier products).
- Use absorbent products that keep the urine away from the skin.
- If you stay in bed a lot or sit in a chair most of the day, protect your skin from moisture and do not lie on any areas that are open or have a rash.
- If you are caring for someone who does not move, turn them frequently and support them in different positions by using pillows or wedges.

The skin is usually slightly acidic. The acidic pH is a major factor that helps prevent the invasion of the skin by bacteria, particularly yeast and fungus. This is often referred to as the "protective acid mantle" of the skin. Furthermore, the presence of excessive skin surface moisture contributes to the growth of bacteria that can lead to skin breakdown and infection. When combined with changes in skin pH into the alkaline range, the effect is particularly devastating.

An alkaline pH also adversely affects the skin, further enhancing the loss of normal skin integrity in the person whose skin is already compromised by exposure to urine and feces. When skin is subject to moisture from urine in combination with fecal matter, further skin trauma is produced when the urea (from the urine) is broken down into ammonia by bacteria in the stool. All of these factors work in concert to weaken the skin. Weakened skin, in turn, is more susceptible to irritation, breakdown, and further problems.

Proper use of soaps, skin products, topical antimicrobials (agents which inhibit the growth of germs), gentle pH balanced skin cleansers, and appropriate barrier products help wash away urinary and fecal matter and prevent skin breakdown. No-rinse perineal washes and cleansers are more skin friendly than most bar soaps because they are convenient, timesaving, and effectively remove urine and/or feces without patient discomfort. These cleansers are also preferable to the popular bar soaps because the cleaning agents and antiseptics used in these formulations are gentler to the skin. Additionally, no-rinse perineal cleansers are pH balanced for the skin, whereas bar soaps are almost always in the alkaline range. Some perineal cleansers are also formulated with topical antimicrobials that may decrease the bacteria on the skin.

Creams, ointments, and pastes are skin barriers. However, the recent advent of clear, solvent-based film-forming skin protectants are an even better alternative then creams, ointments, and pastes. Film-forming skin protectants are acrylate-based copolymers that quickly evaporate when applied to the skin, leaving the copolymer behind to form a protective film. This clear film allows for air flow but is impervious to external moisture and skin irritants.

Careful and close attention to skin care reduces the occurrence of skin breakdown in persons with incontinence.

Dave is a seventy-year-old man who has been bedridden for the past five years. He is cared for by his daughter, Becky. Dave has urge incontinence and often urinates without any warning. His daughter finds him wet before she can offer him the urinal. Becky managed her father's problem by wrapping blue pads around his penis and placing several blue pads underneath him on the bed. Lately his visiting nurse has noted an ever-increasing red area on his scrotum. She suggested a condom catheter, but Becky could never get the device to stay on because her father's penis was retracted. The visiting nurse fears that the reddened area on his scrotum will progress to a bedsore and has suggested more aggressive management of his incontinence. She advised Becky to wash her father's perineum, penis, scrotum, and buttocks with a perineal wash and to apply a protective skin barrier product after washing him in the morning. The nurse also suggested that Becky use cloth underpads and an incontinence brief to manage her father's incontinence. Since starting the skin care program, Dave's skin has improved dramatically.

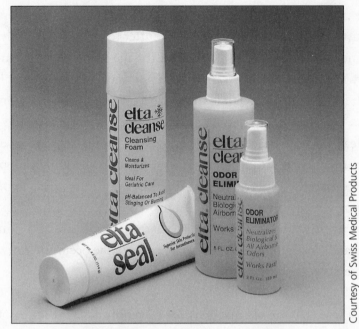

Courtesy of Swiss Medical Products

Figure 17.13 Cleansing foam odor eliminators

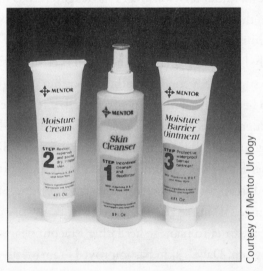

Courtesy of Mentor Urology

Figure 17.14 Moisture cream, skin cleanser, barrier ointment

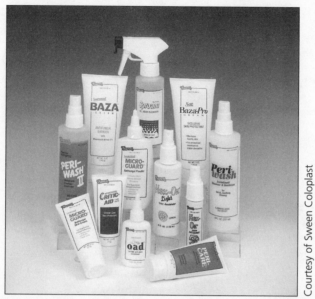

Courtesy of Sween Coloplast

Figure 17.15 Moisturizers, perineal cleansers, barrier skin ointment

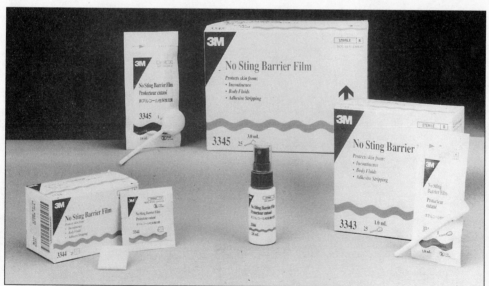

Courtesy of 3M

Figure 17.16 No-sting barrier film

CHAPTER 18

PELVIC PROLAPSE AND
SUPPORT DEVICES

As women age, the tissues that support pelvic organs may become overly stretched, causing the pelvic organs to drop and sometimes protrude through the vaginal opening. This is called *prolapse*.

PELVIC ORGAN
SUPPORT DEVICES

Women with prolapse have poor pelvic support, allowing the vagina, uterus, and rectum to descend (drop) below their normal positions. Loss of support in this area will cause stress UI. There are five kinds of prolapse: urethrocele, cystocele, uterine prolapse, rectocele, and enterocele. They are defined as follows:

1. Urethrocele: Descent of the lower part of the urethra into the vagina.
2. Cystocele: Tissue between the bladder and the vagina has lost its tone and allows the bladder to protrude (drop) down into the vagina. Like a hernia, the cystocele can become worse with time.

3. Uterine prolapse: Descent of the uterus and cervix into the vagina.
4. Rectocele: Protrusion of the rectal wall into the vagina.
5. Enterocele: Descent of the small intestine from the vagina. May occur in women whose uterus has been removed.

There are three grades of prolapse:

Grade 1: The prolapse bulges toward the opening of the vagina.
Grade 2: The prolapse is at the opening of the vagina.
Grade 3: The prolapse protrudes or drops out of the vagina.

The most severe form of prolapse is when the vagina and uterus protrude completely outside the body; this is called *procidentia*.

In prolapse cases, women may find that they have to empty their bladders often or have unwanted urine leakage. Women with a cystocele or uterine prolapse may complain of urinary urgency and frequency, describe a dripping or bulging feeling in their vaginas, or feel as though they are sitting on a tennis ball. Childbirth, heavy lifting, chronic straining during bowel movements, and loss of estrogen may contribute to pelvic prolapse.

An operation can correct pelvic prolapse, especially cystocele. However, an optimal treatment for prolapse is the use of a mechanical device called a pessary. The word *pessary* can be found in both Greek and Latin literature. Mechanical devices have been reported since the time of Hippocrates, who mentioned the use of fruit (a pomegranate) placed in the vagina to support a prolapse.

Use of a pessary is an excellent treatment for supporting pelvic organ prolapse. It has been found that by placing a pessary into the vagina, incontinence symptoms can be relieved. A pessary looks like a contraceptive diaphragm, but the outside rim is hard. Like a diaphragm, it is put into the vagina and rests against the cervix, lifting and supporting the pelvic organs (see Figure 18.1). More than 200 different types of pessaries have been invented, but only a few are used today.

Pessaries come in many shapes, but are usually round. Cube- or U-shaped ones are also available. You should not be able to feel the pessary when it is placed inside you. A pessary must be frequently removed, at least during the first month of use. This can be done by your doctor, nurse, or yourself. An estrogen cream should always be prescribed for use with a pessary and patients should be instructed about pessary removal, cleansing, and reinsertion.

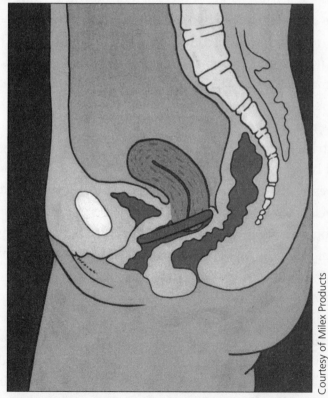

Courtesy of Milex Products

Fligure 18.1 Ring with support pessary in position

In the past, pessaries were used to treat not only pelvic relaxation but also malposition of the uterus, incompetent (weak) cervix, dysmenorrhea (difficult and painful menses), and menstrual irregularities.

Most complications associated with pessaries are minor. Improper fit is common; it takes time and patience to fit pessaries, particularly in older women. Chronic irritation, erosion of the vagina, ulceration of the vagina, and vaginal fistulas (openings in the walls of the vagina) can occur in women who do not properly care for the pessary or who do not go for regular follow-up visits with their practitioner. If ulceration and abrasion of the vaginal wall occur, the pessary should be changed to a smaller size. Adverse effects include back pain, foul-smelling vaginal discharge, or bleeding. Leukorrhea (white discharge from the vagina) is probably the most common problem associated with pessary use, due to the presence of a foreign object in the vagina. Urinary retention can result if the pessary compresses the urethra into the pubic bone.

The optimal method of care for the vagina or the frequency of pessary removal differs from woman to woman. Lubrication of either the pessary or the vagina is usually necessary prior to insertion. Pressure should be applied toward the back, and the device should be placed high in the vagina. The pessary should be removed and cleaned at least every three months, depending upon the presence and amount of discharge, type of pessary, and the patient's comfort level. Not all women are able or willing to insert the pessary themselves. Estrogen cream may be prescribed before a pessary is fitted to prevent ulceration and breakdown of the vaginal tissue. Women with a history of cancer, which precludes the use of estrogen, can use other creams or moisturizers on a daily or weekly basis.

Many medical providers, especially nurse practitioners, have had success using pessaries in carefully selected patients. Women report improved continence and ambulation with their use; personal care is made easier and hygiene improved. In the last few years, pessaries have become more popular for use in elderly women. As the population of American women ages, the prevalence of significant pelvic organ prolapse will rise. The use of pessaries may represent an alternative for frail elders who are not candidates for other therapies.

Types of Pessaries

The pessaries that are available today are very effective for premenopausal women with first- to second-degree prolapse. Elderly women with large vaginal vaults and third-degree and greater prolapse usually have a difficult time retaining the pessaries currently on the market. Unfortunately, these women are usually poor surgical candidates, so a well-fitting pessary is the best alternative. The most commonly used pessaries (see Figure 18.2) are:

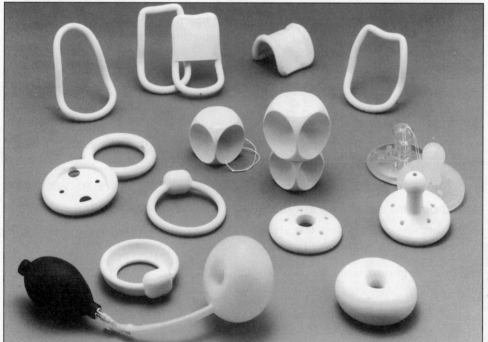

Courtesy of Milex Products

Figure 18.2 Types of pessaries

- Smith Hodge—used most often for a retroverted (tipped to the back) uterus in younger women.
- Ring—useful in cases of first- and second-degree uterine prolapse.
- Ring with support—designed especially for uterine prolapse associated with a mild cystocele.
- Doughnut—useful for third-degree prolapse.
- Cube—effective in some elderly patients where there is markedly decreased vaginal tone.
- Gellhorn—supplied in a rigid, acrylic form and a flexible form. This is one of the most common pessaries used for third-degree prolapse or procidentia.
- Gehrung—an archlike U-shaped pessary which is designed to raise the bladder floor and thin out a rectocele. It is also used with a cystocele.
- Shaatz—used for mild cystocele and prolapse.
- Incontinence dish and ring—modified pessaries recommended for stress UI with mild prolapse. These pessaries were recently introduced and provide support for the prolapse at the bladder-urethra junction, thus preventing stress UI.

Doctors or nurses who routinely see women and are likely to make assessments of pelvic organ prolapse through pelvic examination are more likely to prescribe a pessary. These clinicians will readily prescribe and fit this device. Nurse practitioners have seen an increase in the use of pessaries in homebound persons and those residing in nursing homes.

Prescribing a pessary is largely a function of an individual physician's or nurse's experience and training. A pessary is fitted individually for each woman and must be comfortable. Usually, the clinician obtains the pessary and through trial and error attempts to fit the woman using various sizes and types. The cost of the pessary is usually around $38 and is partially covered by Medicare and other insurers.

When wearing a pessary, a woman should call her doctor or nurse if there is any vaginal discharge, itching, foul odor, or pain, inability to urinate or empty the bladder or have bowel movements, or back pain. You do not need to douche when using a pessary, but if you have a discharge (drainage) from your vagina, a vinegar and water douche might help to make the pessary more comfortable and less irritating. Trimo-san, an antibacterial ointment, is a useful product.

A pessary can remain in place for several months as long as it is removed and cleaned regularly. Problems are unusual, but can occur if the pessary is misused or forgotten. Ulceration (tearing of the wall) of the vagina and fistula (opening between the rectum and vagina) formation are common problems. Women who are pregnant, have a vaginal infection, or who have had recent vaginal surgery should not use a pessary. The ring and Gehrung pessaries can be worn during sex, depending on comfort.

TAKING OUT
YOUR PESSARY

1. Empty your bladder.
2. Find the position that is easiest for removing it. Usually women lie down, squat on a toilet, or lift one leg.
3. Put two fingers in your vagina and grab the pessary, slowly turning it as you pull it down and out.
4. Wash the pessary with soap and warm water. Then dry it.

BLADDER SUPPORT PROSTHESIS

Marie was a very active lady who planned conferences and dinner meetings for small companies. She had been suffering with stress incontinence for several years. She would leak urine when she coughed, someone hugged her, or even when she walked. Her problem caused anxiety and despair, and many times she didn't want to get out of bed because of depression over her problem. She had searched for many solutions. Marie had bladder surgery two years ago in New York City. The surgery was supposed to have cured her, but within six months the incontinence returned. She had been through a course of biofeedback therapy without success. She came to see the continence nurse practitioner to participate in a FDA study on a new device that supported the bladder.

The device Marie was given is the Introl, a removable bladder neck support prosthesis. This prosthesis (an artificial replacement for a body part or organ) is a flexible silicone device that is placed in the vagina to give support to the bladder neck and urethra (see Figure 18.3). It is flexible, ring shaped, and has two rounded prongs at one end.

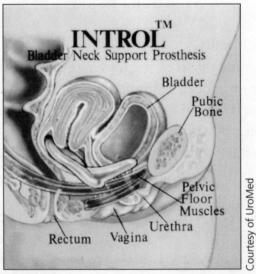

Figure 18.3 Introl™ bladder neck support prosthesis

The prongs elevate (support) the bladder, similar to a surgical procedure. It eliminates surgery, a stay in the hospital, and the need to go through a period of recovery. This device is designed for women who have mild to severe stress incontinence. It may hold promise for women with sufficient manual dexterity who have the ability to learn to insert and remove the device. The device is not for women with vaginal prolapse beyond the vaginal opening or vaginitis, or those who cannot easily remove or insert the device. The Introl comes in many different sizes, and a doctor or nurse will fit you with the proper size. The device is designed to be inserted, removed, washed, and lubricated daily. Problems which can occur with Introl use include irritation in the vagina or vaginal discharge (drainage), but these are rare. This is a very comfortable device to use and is paid for by most insurers.

As soon as the Introl device was positioned correctly against the base of Marie's bladder, her urinary incontinence stopped. She has been using the device for a year and she is 100 percent dry.

CHAPTER 19

TOILETS, COMMODES,
AND COLLECTION DEVICES

What this country needs is a chicken in every pot, a toilet in every house, and a good five-cent cigar.

—VICE PRESIDENT ANDREW H. HIGGINS
IN A SPEECH BEFORE CONGRESS, 1824

Vice President Higgins could not have anticipated the aging population boom of the next century; every house is going to need more than one toilet and that toilet may not be the kind we use today.

COLLECTION
DEVICES

Collection devices "catch" urine. These devices include portable or bedside commodes, urinals, and bedpans which you can use as a toilet when the toilet is either not available or impossible to use.

COMMODE
CHAIR

One way to decrease urine leakage on the way to the bathroom is to make toileting easier. A portable commode chair may be the answer. Some have drop arms and adjustable heights to allow for individual needs. There are also wooden rather than metal commodes that are disguised as easy chairs. When selecting a commode, the following should be considered:

- Height and weight of the person using the commode.
- Mobility and dexterity, especially if the person will need to empty and clean the commode.
- Cost. Most insurers will pay for at least one portable commode per person when a physician writes a letter of medical necessity.

BATHROOM
ARCHITECTURE

Changes in bathroom architecture can also help you remain continent. Removing the bathroom door and using a curtain or swinging doors makes access by a wheelchair possible. Grab bars in the right spot and a toilet seat adapter make the toilet safer. At least one grab bar should run parallel to the floor at a height of 33 inches. Gravity-assisted door-closer mechanisms for the bathroom are helpful. If you are redesigning your bathroom to make toileting easier, recommended dimensions are a minimum of 5' × 5' ×, 5' × 8'. Many people cannot open bathroom doors, because they are unable to grasp and turn the doorknob. In this case, replace doorknobs with lever-type devices or disable the door so that the door opens and closes with a push.

BEDSIDE COMMODES

Bedside commodes (portable commodes) are movable toilets that are wonderful for persons living in their homes or for residents in nursing homes. A bedside commode can be placed close to the bed for easy use at night, or used as a convenient floor toilet when a multistory house does not have a bathroom on every level. If you can get out of bed to urinate, a commode is a better alternative than a bedpan. Bedside commodes are lightweight and easy to maneuver, yet have solid construction. You can buy or rent one from a surgical supply store. It is important that the commode be emptied and the bucket cleaned after every use. To minimize odor and make cleaning the bucket easier, keep water mixed with a disinfectant in the bucket at all times. To camouflage the commode, you can cover it with an attractive cloth or place it behind a screen.

RAISED TOILET SEAT

A raised toilet seat, attached over an existing seat, makes getting up and down much easier, thus allowing for self-toileting. Seats with grab bars on either side are most often recommended to prevent falling and to aid rising.

URINAL

A handheld urinal is a bottle-shaped container with handles that can have two different types of necks. Urinals are useful for people with severe mobility restrictions, particularly when visiting places with inaccessible rest rooms, trav-

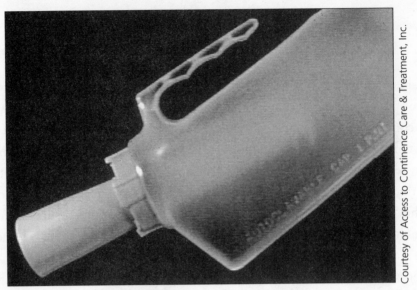

Figure 19.1 Male spillproof urinal

eling, or when confined to bed. They can be placed next to you, can be hung on a bedrail, wheelchair, or walker, or can be laid flat on the bed. There are rehab, spillproof male urinals with large funnel openings to deal with a retracted penis (see Figure 19.1). Often these rehab urinals have flat bottoms so that they can be placed on the bed. The openings in rehab urinals have a flange that extends into the urinal and does not allow backflow even when held almost upside down. Female urinals are a good alternative for persons traveling, sitting in wheelchairs or chairs, or who are bedridden (see Figures 19.2 and 19.3). However, female urinals that work well are not easy to find.

The following should be considered when choosing an urinal:

- Material—Lightweight plastic urinals are useful for people who have difficulty lifting. Steel urinals are very heavy and cumbersome.
- Handles—If grip is a problem, rubber around the handle will add extra

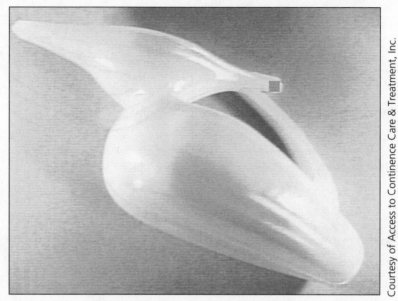

Figure 19.2 Female spillproof urinal

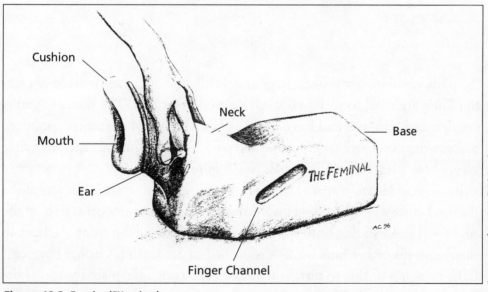

Figure 19.3 Feminal™ urinal

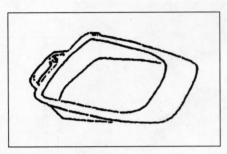
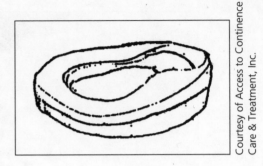

Courtesy of Access to Continence Care & Treatment, Inc.

Figure 19.4 Bedpans

holding power. An extended handle may help if wrist movement is restricted.

- Ease of use and cleaning.
- Spillproof design.

BEDPANS

Bedpans come in many sizes, large and small, and are usually made of plastic. They are used to toilet yourself on a chair or bed. The fracture pan is smaller, easier to use, and has a grip handle. The use of a fracture pan often makes urination more comfortable and pain free for women, especially after surgery for a fracture or hip repair (see Figure 19.4).

It is a good idea to warm a bedpan by running warm water inside and along the rim before use. Sprinkling on a little talcum powder or cornstarch on the edges will make sliding onto the bedpan easier. The person using the bedpan should lift his or her hips while it is pushed underneath his or her buttocks. If the person is unable to turn, roll him or her to one side, place the top of the bedpan (the rounded seat area) against the top of the buttocks below the tailbone, and then assist the person in rolling onto the bedpan. He or she should be positioned over the middle of the bedpan so it won't tip.

INFLATABLE BEDPANS

A U-shaped cushion made of soft, breathable, and washable fabric inflates and elevates the person's buttocks and pelvis 3 to 4 inches above the bed surface (see Figure 19.5). A rubber foot pump or small compact electric air pump is used to inflate the cushion. After the person's buttocks are elevated, a specially designed bedpan is easily inserted between the person's legs. This product is good for the person who is in pain or is difficult to turn and move into position on a bedpan. The product also makes it possible to accomplish treatments and procedures in the perineal area. A waterproof breathable nylon base attached to the inflatable product protects bed linens from soilage.

OTHER DEVICES

PERINEAL PATCH

The perineal or barrier patch is worn over the urethral meatus, outside the opening to the urethra in women (see Figure 19.6). The patch is disposable and is about the size of a quarter. The patch has an adhesive coating that is placed over the meatus to form a seal that stops urine from leaking. The patch will fall off when the woman voids. The device is helpful for women with mild stress incontinence, those who leak urine when they cough, sneeze, laugh, or those who play certain sports. The patch is available by prescription.

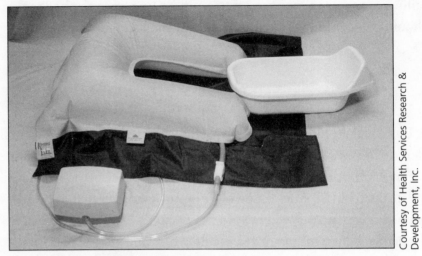

Figure 19.5 Kimbro Pelvic Lift™

Courtesy of Health Services Research & Development, Inc.

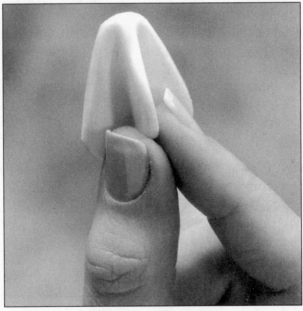

Figure 19.6 Perineal patch

Courtesy of UroMed

URINARY CONTROL INSERT

The urinary control insert is a soft and flexible, catheter-like device that is inserted into the urethra. The urinary insert is a single-use device designed for women and is about one-fifth the size of a tampon. It is held in place by a small balloon which is inflated with air using a syringe. The device is inserted into the urethra using a special applicator (syringe). Once in place, the insert blocks the flow of urine (see Figure 19.7). Whenever the woman needs to urinate, she removes the device with a small string which deflates the balloon. The insert can be worn for no more than six hours at a time. The urinary control insert is available by prescription.

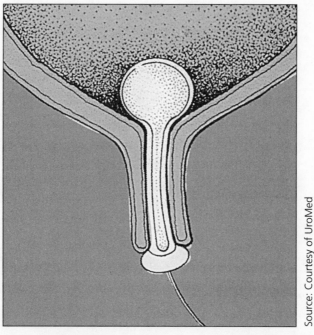

Source: Courtesy of UroMed

Figure 19.7 Reliance® urinary control insert

Vacuum Suction Product

Newer collection devices are still being developed for the very ill, frail person. One such product for women that wicks the urine away through a suction pump is available. This device combines a perineal pad and suction to remove urine and store it in a compartment that can later be emptied. When the urine from an incontinence episode hits the perineal pad, tubes in the pad whisk the urine into the storage compartment, keeping the person's perineal area dry at all times. The perineal pad should be changed at least three times daily. This device has been used successfully for persons who are living at home, bedridden, and need total care. In these cases, other product or management options have failed or are not appropriate, and this system has been a lifesaver for caregivers.

CHAPTER 20

THE CAREGIVING DILEMMA: GROWING OLD WITH INCONTINENCE

The elderly population is skyrocketing as baby boomers age. By the year 2020, more than one in six Americans will be aged sixty-five or older. The fastest-growing group will be the old-old, people aged eighty-five and older, whose numbers will more than double from the current level. This aging population is already demanding better solutions to the health care problems they face. One of those problems is urinary incontinence.

HELPING A FAMILY MEMBER WITH INCONTINENCE

Mr. G's family members brought him to the continence specialist's office because they couldn't deal with his stubborn refusal to wear Depends®. Mr. G. is eighty-six, suffered a stroke six months ago, and has weakness in his left side. Before the stroke, Mr. G. had some prostate problems that caused him to urinate frequently. The family reports that Mr. G. loses urine without warning. He is so embarrassed that he has stopped visiting his friends at the corner diner and no longer goes to the senior center for lunch. The family has put pressure on him to wear Depends® so he can go out of the house.

Table 20.1 The Demographics of Caregiving

Chances are that in the next century you will be in the position of caring for a family member who has a problem with incontinence. Consider the following:

Where do older people live?

- 43 percent have lived in their present homes for over twenty years.
- Almost 30 percent live alone (32 percent of women, 22 percent of men).
- Thirty-three percent of men and 50 percent of women over age sixty-five who are widowed, separated, or divorced live with adult children or other family members.

Who provides care in the home?

- Nearly 80 percent of primary caregivers are women, who provide the majority of hands-on care such as changing incontinence products, catheters, and so on. Daughters outnumber sons three to one.
- One-third of caregivers are age sixty-five and older.
- Women today can expect to spend eighteen years of their lives helping an aging parent and seventeen years caring for children.
- Fifty-three percent of caregivers report they are caring for someone with urinary incontinence.

Who lives in nursing homes?

- Less than 5 percent of those aged sixty-five and older live in nursing homes, but more than 25 percent will be in a nursing home at some point during their later years.
- Over 70 percent of nursing home residents are women.
- Almost 10 percent of older people living in private homes would require nursing home placement if family support were withdrawn.
- At least 50 percent of nursing home residents have urinary incontinence; 48 percent have fecal incontinence.
- If you go into a nursing home continent, you have a 39 percent chance of being incontinent by two weeks after admission.

Adapted from: Lustbader, W. and Hooyman, N. R., *Taking Care of Aging Family Members*, New York: The Free Press, 1994.

Recently Mr. G. was taken to the emergency room because he was dehydrated—he had stopped drinking water and juice so he wouldn't wet as much. His family members are frustrated and angry with Mr. G, and they want to know if they should put him in a nursing home.

Mr. G. is not unusual. Men with urinary incontinence seem to be more finicky than women about being away from home. Men who must wear disposable diapers or undergarments can't easily hide spare diapers in a large purse or bag. Men are embarrassed when they have to change their diapers or pads and deposit soiled ones in the trash in front of other men in public rest rooms. On the other hand, public ladies' rooms have small garbage cans in each stall for feminine hygiene product disposal.

For persons living at home or in a nursing home, incontinence can be a significant burden, since they are dependent on others for their care. Assessment and treatment of incontinence for persons who are frail, have dementia, or have physical impairments are somewhat different than for those who are well and able to practice self-care. Treatment options are limited for the impaired. A family caregiver (or professional) is most often responsible for carrying out the treatment plan or management strategies.

To make any impact on incontinence and its management in older adults, it is important that caregivers have a clear view about it. Effective caregivers must understand the problem of incontinence. Caregivers should:

- Understand the physical and emotional distress that may result from an untreated urinary control problem.
- Demonstrate an understanding of incontinence as a symptom.
- Consistently reinforce positive behavior.
- Understand that success with rehabilitative behavioral treatments can occur.

HOME CARE SERVICES

More and more people are living into their eighties, nineties, and even over one hundred! Many still live in their own homes, do their own cooking, and (for better or worse) drive their own cars. It's only human to want to stay in familiar surroundings, remain involved in community activities, and participate in family gatherings until the end of our days. Unfortunately, it is not always possible to maintain that independence. Unforeseen illness or disability and natural aging processes force many to seek physical care. When this situation arises, most people want to stay in their own home and receive the needed care. That is why home care is the fastest-growing segment of the health care industry. The number of families providing long-term care to disabled and older relatives is expected to increase substantially in the next few decades. Financially, home care is a better option than nursing home care; it can be provided at lower cost because the burden of caregiving lies with immediate and extended family members. As you become less independent, it is most likely that you'll be taken care of by a family member, probably your wife, daughter, daughter-in-law, or niece, since 75 percent of chronic home care is handled by women. Partners and spouses are the most common caregivers. Adult children and other family members usually only assume care responsibilities when a partner is absent.

Sources of Help for Family Caregivers

If you find yourself in a situation where you will be responsible for or actually providing the care for a family member, you will need to identify resources to assist you in that caregiving. Look in the phone book for your local Area Agency on Aging (AAA), an organization which has information on programs for the elderly. AAAs are located in all rural and urban communities in the United States and provide federally mandated programs which furnish nonmedical services (for example, transportation, home-delivered meals, and so on) from resources based within the community. Some AAAs have a case manager, usually a social worker, who can assist you in finding and accessing services and professionals to help with your caregiving. Local home health care agencies or visiting nurse agencies are also excellent medical caregiving resources.

Home health care is divided into custodial (supportive) and skilled services. Custodial care is not covered under Medicare when it is the only kind of care needed. Medicare covers skilled care if the person is homebound and it is ordered by a physician. In addition to registered nurses, home care agencies provide home health aides, companions, and physical therapists. Home health aides (HHAs) assist with personal care for people with health problems, similar to nurse's aides in hospitals and nursing homes. If the physician determines that your family member needs skilled care, Medicare and other insurance companies will pay for the services of an HHA. HHA fees vary, but can range from $10 to $20 per hour.

There are community-based social services for elders who need to get out and interact with others and for family members who need a break from caregiving. The most common places are senior centers. A senior center is similar to a club where older people can gather, eat meals, meet friends, and attend planned programs. Senior centers are usually free, except for a lunch charge. Another type of center is an adult day care center. These centers provide a safe, structured environment for frail at-risk elders. They may provide services such as bathing, rehabilitative programs, and even a place for napping. Many family members who care for elder relatives bring them to a day care center during working hours. This is especially helpful for incontinent persons, as some adult day care centers can handle incontinence care, especially toileting schedules. Fees range from $20 to $80 per day. Respite care programs are available when you need a break from caregiving. Elders are able to stay overnight at these facilities and total care is provided at a rate of about $100 per day.

Is Incontinence a Problem?

As a concerned spouse or relative, how can you tell if your partner or family member is hiding an incontinence problem? There are a few questions that may guide you:

- Is your family member unwilling to be away from home for more than one or two hours?
- Is there a sudden change in your family member's activity level?
- Do you smell urine in your family member's house or on his or her clothes?
- When your family member arrives at your house or at his or her destination, does he or she rush to the bathroom?
- Does your family member resist taking off a coat, suit jacket, or long sweater in public?
- Does your family member resist sitting down in social settings or sit "funny" in a chair?
- Does your family member purchase feminine hygiene pads even after menopause?

If the answer to any of these questions is yes, you should talk with other family members about your suspicions of a urinary incontinence problem. Then seek assistance from a doctor, nurse, social worker, or other medical professional.

A couple may maintain a taboo against discussing incontinence, despite their mutual awareness of the problem. A partner may be repelled by the stench on clothing and upholstery, yet say nothing in order to avoid humiliating the incontinent partner. A partner who refuses to perpetuate the silence and instead confides in family members may feel guilty for violating the other person's trust. However, once an incontinent partner becomes ill, necessitating home caregiving, the incontinence may become unbearable to both partners.

Incontinence is a relentless source of weariness for caregivers, especially elderly ones. Physical exertion, often called caregiver burden, increases day by day. The ill person needs to be lifted and turned to prevent skin breakdown, to change incontinence products and bedpads, and to wash away urine. And incontinence is not only a daytime problem. During the night, a caregiver's sleep is disturbed to assist with toileting activities. There are situations where the caregiver's burden is so great that the caregiver becomes ill and, in the case of an elderly frail partner, may even die before the incontinent person being cared for. Not all persons living at home are dependent on caregivers for their toileting needs. Many elders are frail but can still get to the bathroom on their own. Choosing the correct product or device to assist the person in maintaining their toileting independence should be the goal of the spouse or family member. Simple changes in the home environment can guarantee that the person can independently manage his or her toileting needs.

Denial of incontinence by an older family member can be a tricky dilemma for both family members and professionals who may be assisting the family with caregiving. Older persons lose a degree of smell sensitivity as they age, and some block out their awareness of their incontinence problem to avoid its implications. If other family members confront the denial head-on, they may provoke hostility and humiliation and cause an incontinent individual to withdraw further from acknowledging the problem.

If you are caring for a family member at home who is basically immobile and bedridden, that person does not necessarily have to be incontinent. If getting out of bed to use the bathroom or bedside commode is not feasible, then offer a bedpan or urinal. Toileting is a private and personal act, so you need to be aware of the need for some privacy.

The tips listed in Table 20.2 may assist you in toileting a family member.

Table 20.2 Tips to Promote Safe and Independent Toileting

- Try to give the person a private bathroom so it's never being used by someone else. If a bathroom is inaccessible, use a bedside commode, urinal, or bedpan.

- Keep the bed height sufficient so when the person sits on the edge of the bed, feet are flat and the person can easily accomplish going from sitting to standing.

- Keep a clear, direct walking path to the toilet.

- Place night-lights along the path to bathroom.

- Make sure your family member can easily use the toilet; provide raised toilet seat, grab bars, and so on.

- Make sure your family member wears clothing that is easy to remove.

- Make sure the person empties his or her bladder before going to bed.

- Locate the bathroom when traveling or carry a portable urinal. Choose seats in restaurants and theaters that are near a bathroom.

- Use underpads (reusable or disposable) under bedsheets, on chairs, and in the car. Avoid use of garbage bags, rubber pads, or shower liners as these may be too slippery or irritate skin.

- Open windows or use deodorizers to cut down on odors. (A cut-up onion in a room will absorb odors without leaving its own smell. Also, an open box of baking soda will reduce odors.)

NIGHTTIME INCONTINENCE

Night incontinence can be a particular problem, especially if family members must get up to assist with toileting. Efforts should be made to maximize the sleep period. Sleep patterns change with age and become more fragmented. There is a decreased amount of deep sleep (stages 3 and 4) and higher percentage of stage 1 sleep. Therefore, sleep occurs for shorter periods with many wakenings. To help the person minimize night voidings, follow these measures:

- Restrict fluids in the evening: Have the person drink the majority of fluids before 6 P.M., but spread the fluids throughout the day.
- Eliminate all caffeine and alcohol-containing foods and fluids, especially from the evening meal.
- Increase urine output during the day: By taking a one-to-two-hour nap with legs elevated to level of the heart, the person will increase urine output during the day, thus decreasing output and need to void during the night.

INCONTINENCE IN THE NURSING HOME

A RED FLAG FOR NURSING HOME PLACEMENT: BURDENSOME INCONTINENCE

The family members of a person with urinary incontinence may eventually decide that caregiving is too burdensome and the person can no longer live at home. They may search for an alternative living arrangement that usually involves some form of community or group living. In many cases, caregivers will choose a nursing home for their incontinent family members. UI is often the problem which precipitates or contributes to a person's decision to enter a nursing home or to a family's decision to place an elder family member into nursing home care.

ALTERNATIVE LIVING POSSIBILITIES

Alternative living arrangements have broadened over the last ten years. Individuals with incontinence are now accepted into assisted living situations if they can manage their own incontinence. Table 20.3 outlines the specific assisted living categories.

There are nearly 2 million nursing home residents in the United States. Urinary incontinence is a common and expensive problem in nursing home residents. There are many reasons for the problem of urinary incontinence in nursing homes. Restricted mobility is an important factor, as nursing home residents who are placed in restraints or in wheelchairs are unable to toilet when needed. Social indifference or mental incompetence also plays a role in the incidence of incontinence in nursing homes.

When Carolyn visits her grandmother in Shady Pines Nursing Home, she often finds her sitting in urine or stool. Carolyn is disturbed because Grandma was always a meticulously clean person when she lived at home. At home, Grandma was able to make it to the commode, if it was close to her bed or chair. Grandma knows when she has to void, but she thinks the nurses prefer that she go in her diapers, that's why she has them on. Carolyn has discussed this with her grandmother, who says she doesn't want to be a bother to the staff because they are so busy with other residents who really need help. Grandma says it's hard to go to the toilet on someone else's schedule. Also, she gets the urge suddenly, and it's so strong that the staff would never get to her in time.

As you can see by Carolyn's experience, caregiving doesn't end when your family member enters a nursing home. It's just another phase of caregiving. It's still emotionally draining and still requires family involvement. In 1989 the United States government developed uniform federal standards for every

Table 20.3 Alternative Living Situations

CATEGORY	DEFINITION
Retirement communities	Self-contained for older persons who want to live with others their age.
Continuous-care retirement communities	Retirement communities that provide continuous care for the resident's lifetime, including nursing home care.
Senior housing	Usually federal, state, or local government–financed and supported housing designed for older persons. Most often a middle-income housing program.
Board and care homes	A home that is a small, friendly arrangement for persons who need help with personal care. Most homes will provide assistance with bathing, dressing, and toileting.
Assisted living	Housing complex that provides several services for the 30 to 100 elderly who need minimal assistance with tasks such as dressing and some supervision.
Adult foster care	A family will care for an elder in its own home. Help with bathing, dressing, and other personal needs usually is provided.
Home sharing	Social service agencies may have a program of roommate-matching for seniors.
Nursing home	Skilled nursing care is provided around the clock. Also intermediate care for persons who can participate in some independent care.

Adapted from: Rob, C., *The Caregivers Guide*, Boston: Houghton Mifflin Company, 1991.

aspect of nursing home life, including the treatment of urinary incontinence. These regulations have brought a new philosophy based on two very important requirements—the nursing home must provide quality care and it must consider the individual resident's quality of life.

Many people enter a nursing home continent but lose their ability to use the toilet soon afterward, usually because they are in a strange environment and the staff fails to take them to the bathroom regularly. Are you unsure about the quality of care in a particular nursing home? Sometimes the smells tell the real story. Staff attitudes toward incontinence play a major role in the way UI residents are treated. Staff may act out negative feelings toward these residents. Staff may also avoid residents or ignore their needs. Ninety percent of the actual care, bathing, dressing, and feeding is provided by nurse assistants, who have limited training and education in the care of older adults.

A continence nurse practitioner conducted an in-service program on urinary incontinence for all staff members on the day shift of a large nursing home facility. The continence specialist nurse practitioner gave an overview of urinary incontinence, age-related changes that occur in the bladder, and treatments that are successful with nursing home residents. During the in-service the nurse practitioner emphasized that incontinence also occurs in young adult women, especially during pregnancy. The nurse specialist asked the staff to tell about their experiences with residents who have incontinence. A nurse's assistant, Joanie, stated that she feels that sometimes residents are wetting to "get to her." The specialist asked the assistant who gets more attention in the home—the wet resident or the dry resident? The answer was, "Of course, the wet resident." So if a resident is lonely, depressed, and seeking attention, wouldn't urinary incontinence be an option? The staff felt it would be. The specialist stressed that the behavior that is expected should be rewarded. Most residents are incontinent for reasons other than for seeking attention. At the end of the in-service, a charge nurse on the unit told the nurse practitioner in private that every time she lifted a resident she leaked enough urine to saturate a panty liner. The nurse admitted that because of her incontinence problem, she tried to avoid lifting residents.

The feelings that Joanie expressed are shared by many nursing home staff— that residents are seeking secondary gains by being incontinent. The incontinent resident may perceive that the only way to get attention, although many times negative attention, is by being incontinent. Staff members believe that incontinence is expected in nursing home residents, as UI is a natural part of aging, and convey their acceptance of incontinence to nursing home residents. Staff members also feel that it's quicker to change an incontinence pad than it is to toilet a resident. The hopeless acceptance of incontinence can make it into a nonproblem. However, good care in nursing homes means that residents are regularly toileted by staff according to an individualized care plan that has a specific schedule. Staff should also toilet a resident upon request.

Since 1990, the Minimum Data Set (MDS), a standardized screening and assessment form, is required by the Health Care Financing Administration (HCFA) for reimbursement. The MDS must be completed on all residents at admission, quarterly, and when a significant change occurs in medical status. See page 279 for the continence section of the MDS. According to the Resident Assessment Protocol (RAP) issued by Medicare, all nursing home residents should be systematically and regularly evaluated for incontinence. Consider that the nursing home staff should:

- Assess bladder and bowel function.
- Review medications.
- Observe toileting behavior, including urinary frequency.
- Identify and evaluate the causes of incontinence.
- Determine response to a reminder to void.
- Check for hard stool in the rectum (fecal impaction).
- Look for pelvic prolapse.
- Check urine for infection.
- Make sure the bladder is completely emptying (check for PVR).

Persons who are care dependent and are experiencing urinary incontinence should receive a basic evaluation. That means a bladder record should be completed for at least three days to determine voiding patterns, incontinence episodes, and precipitants of incontinence. These persons should receive at least a modified physical examination and a review of their medical history. An assessment of mobility (ability to walk), mental changes, and the environment in which they live should take place. Time and distance may be barriers to toileting, especially in nursing homes. It is important to observe the resident toileting, as the distance to the toilet is important as well as the time it takes the resident to reach the toilet. Staff should determine if the resident knows the location of the toilet and understands its appropriate use. The use of restraints can cause incontinence since the person is unable to go to the bathroom independently when necessary. The presence of a possible infection and a PVR measurement should also be done. However, urodynamic testing is probably not necessary in this group of individuals unless a urine obstruction is suspected.

If based on the assessment it is determined that the resident's medical problems are severe and bladder retraining is not possible, attention should focus on identifying the product or products that best meet the resident's needs.

If the resident's incontinence is caused by functional barriers, attention should be focused on voiding patterns so toileting programs can be designed. If the resident can be rehabilitated, success may also be achieved with pelvic muscle rehabilitation and bladder retraining. Carolyn's grandmother is a perfect case for retraining. She knows when she has to void, but she can't hold it until the nurses can toilet her. She can be taught bladder retraining—how to control the urge and to do some quick squeezes with her pelvic muscle. That may give her the control and time to wait for a nurse to help her. However, the staff needs to respond promptly to her requests for toileting.

What did the staff do about Allen? Allen had lived at the Salen Nursing Home for two years, ever since his wife died. Allen doesn't have any children or any relatives to speak of and his only visitor is the pastor from the Baptist

SECTION H. CONTINENCE IN LAST 14 DAYS

1. CONTINENCE SELF-CONTROL CATEGORIES
   (Code for resident's performance over all shifts.)

   0. CONTINENT—Complete control (includes use of indwelling urinary catheter or ostomy device that does not leak urine or stool)

   1. USUALLY CONTINENT—BLADDER, incontinent episodes once a week or less; BOWEL, less than weekly

   2. OCCASIONALLY INCONTINENT—BLADDER, 2 or more times a week but not daily; BOWEL, once a week

   3. FREQUENTLY INCONTINENT—BLADDER, tended to be incontinent daily, but some control present (e.g., on day shift); BOWEL, 2–3 times a week

   4. INCONTINENT—Had inadequate control. BLADDER, multiple daily episodes; BOWEL, all (or almost all) of the time

a.	BOWEL CONTINENCE	Control of bowel movement, with appliance or bowel continence programs, if employed
b.	BLADDER CONTINENCE	Control of urinary bladder function (if dribbles, volume insufficient to soak through underpants), with appliances (e.g., Foley) or continence programs, if employed

2.	BOWEL ELIMINATION PATTERN	Bowel elimination pattern regular—at least one movement every three days	a.	Diarrhea	c.
				Fecal impaction	d.
		Constipation	b.	**None of the above**	e.

3.	APPLIANCES AND PROGRAMS	Any scheduled toileting plan	a.	Didn't use toilet room/commode/urinal	f.
		Bladder retraining program	b.	Pads, briefs used	g.
		External (condom) catheter	c.	Enemas/irrigation	h.
		Indwelling catheter	d.	Ostomy present	i.
		Intermittent catheter	e.	**None of the above**	j.

4.	CHANGE IN URINARY	Resident's urinary continence has changed as compared to status of 90 days ago (or since last assessment if less

Source: Adapted from *Long-Term Care Facility Assessment Instrument (RAI) User's Manual, Version 2.0,* by J. Morris, K. Murphy, and S. Nonemaker, p. B-6, with permission of the Health Care Financing Administration, © 1995.

church. At times, Allen appears to be depressed. He recently was in the hospital for a heart problem. Since his return, Allen lies in bed most of the day, especially after meals. He may go to physical therapy in the afternoon. Sometimes Allen knows what day it is, but sometimes he gets confused about where he is. Allen has urinary and bowel incontinence and wears a large cloth wraparound diaper. Salen Nursing Home has a continence nurse practitioner who is working with the staff to implement a bladder and bowel retraining program. Allen was the first candidate for the program. The staff checked Allen for a bladder infection and made sure he was emptying his bladder completely. The staff compiled a bladder and bowel diary for three days. The results of the diary showed that Allen usually had a bowel accident mid-morning and urinary incontinence episodes two or three times between 9 A.M. and 7 P.M. The staff had a care plan meeting with the continence practitioner and decided to place Allen on the following toileting schedule:

6:30 A.M. upon awakening
9:00 A.M. after breakfast—encourage Allen to have a bowel movement
11:00 A.M.. before lunch
2:30 P.M. after therapy
5:00 P.M. before dinner
8:00 P.M. before going to bed
11:00 P.M. night shift staff

To make this program successful, the staff was taught prompted voiding techniques. The staff checked Allen at these times and asked him if he was wet or dry. The staff verified his correct answers. If Allen was dry, the staff gave Allen praise and positive reinforcement. For example, the staff told Allen, "Allen, your pad is dry, it's been three hours, that's a long time. You really have control over your bladder." The staff also toileted Allen at the time of checking. The staff stayed with Allen to play a game of checkers, his favorite pastime. *Remember, positive feedback should be given for the behavior that is expected, continence!* If at the time of checking Allen, the staff found his pad wet, the staff toileted Allen and told him to try to be dry at the next scheduled toileting visit.

The staff must still toilet Allen. But in two weeks, Allen had become 100 percent bowel continent and had decreased his urinary incontinent episodes to four or five times per week. The most significant change was that Allen asked to be toileted on a more consistent basis.

Success stories like Allen's are achievable with a caring staff and nursing home administrative support.

If you are planning to put a family member or friend in a nursing home and are unsure about the home's attitude toward the problem of urinary incontinence, ask the following questions of staff members:

- *How do they determine if a resident is incontinent?* The nursing home has a responsibility to identify those who are incontinent and those who are at risk for becoming incontinent. Staff should assess the resident's toileting habits and practices. It is also important to determine the resident's perception of his or her problem.

- *Do they investigate the cause?* The MDS guidelines give nursing home staff a template for investigating causes of incontinence. It is not very different than the evaluation discussed in Chapter 11.

- *Have they developed, implemented, and reviewed appropriate continence management programs?* Experience and research has shown that residents who do not have memory problems usually respond willingly to education and management programs. They want to improve their condition and quality of life.

Significant advances have been seen over the past five years in nursing home management of residents. These advances encompass enhanced quality of all aspects of resident care, including incontinence care. If you are planning to place a family member or friend in a nursing home, investigate that home's approach and philosophy regarding incontinence care.

Chapter 21

MAINTAINING CONTINENCE AND PREVENTING INCONTINENCE

Unfortunately, the general public has little access to information about how to prevent incontinence and maintain continence. Medical professionals and manufacturers of incontinence products do not actively promote self-care practices. Regular toileting and increasing fluid intake, exercise, and weight reduction do contribute to continence but are not explained or encouraged. Research shows that incontinence in the elderly who live at home can be prevented. By increasing the number of women who discuss urinary incontinence with their doctors from the present 41 percent to 71 percent, and by assuming that these women will all perform effective bladder training, cases of incontinence could be reduced by 50,000 each year.

Effective preventive measures need to be identified for those persons at risk for developing incontinence. In certain populations, self-care practices are successful in modifying identified risk factors. These populations include women of childbearing age, men with prostate problems, and persons who have multiple medical problems which cause changes in physical function and memory.

A key objective of the U.S. Department of Health and Human Services' "Healthy People 2000" project is to increase to at least 60 percent the proportion of health care providers of older adults who routinely evaluate people age sixty and older for common medical problems. Although most elderly persons are functional and active, research indicates that the health of nonwhite elders is poorer than white elders. This is particularly significant because the number of ethnic minority elders is growing more rapidly than the number of white elders. This trend will continue over the next fifty years. The disparities of health status among the elderly is a serious medical issue. Health promotion activities are important strategies in tackling these inequities.

Wellness promotion among nonwhite elders in the community requires an unique approach. These groups often value their independence, use folk medicine and self-help remedies, and tend to be more resistant to traditional medical care.

SUCCESS OF ONE
HEALTH PROMOTION PROGRAM

A health promotion project called Dry Expectations™ was conducted in six senior centers in Philadelphia, Pennsylvania, in 1996. The program used self-care practices to improve quality of life for persons experiencing bladder problems. Elder consumers were taught about incontinence and given strategies to prevent the problem. These included good bowel habits, diet changes, and bladder retraining. The project focused on behavioral methods including diet modification, daily self-monitoring of voiding habits, bladder training techniques, bowel management, and the use of absorbent products.

Dry Expectations™ educated two groups: senior center staff members and elder consumers. Selection of a senior center was based on a center's interest in the topic, center location, and specific requirements of the health promotion funding source, the Philadelphia Corporation on Aging, and the area's agency on aging. The project targeted healthy elders who were at risk for developing UI. Subjects were recruited through flyers and posters that were mailed and distributed to specific places in the communities where each site was located. Periodic television and radio public service announcements alerted the target group and its caregivers to the program. To ensure good attendance, sessions were held before lunch, the time of highest attendance at senior centers.

The sessions addressed four areas that affect continence in the elderly:

- Normal function of the urinary tract and age-related changes.
- Bowel irregularity, dietary irritants, and inadequate fluid intake and their impact on the bladder.
- Bladder retraining techniques.
- Absorbent incontinence and skin care products.

In general, the elder consumers rated the sessions very highly, found the program helpful, and almost always recommended it to friends and families. Men seemed comfortable sitting in a predominantly female audience and asked many questions about the prostate. There was confusion from some of the women, who thought that they also had a prostate. Many of the seniors asked if the bladder training could help their grandchildren, who suffered from bed-wetting.

Demonstration of the absorbent products was also well received. Consumers were given samples of various products to use at home. By the end of the sessions, roughly 80 percent of participants felt they had more control over their bladder. The Dry Expectations™ program demonstrates that health promotion programs for incontinence do work! The program is continuing and has expanded to include prostate diseases in men and urinary tract infections and atrophic vaginitis in women.

The Dry Expectations™ model for continence promotion and education is also useful in settings such as women's and men's social groups, breast-feeding classes, health fitness centers, and school health classes—*yes*, school health classes. Grade school children are taught about AIDS and the consequences of unprotected sex. However, most are unaware that their fluid intake is inadequate, that drinking sodas containing caffeine may cause them to urinate more frequently, and that routine exercise helps regulate their bowels. As children move into puberty and young adulthood, this information becomes important for maintenance of their general health. However, bladder health promotion is a serious dilemma. Providers of comprehensive continence services universally agree that the traditional strategies used to encourage people to access medical care are not an effective way to promote continence prevention. Many factors prevent people from seeking out incontinence prevention advice. One of the most common is that self-care methods are readily accepted and used. Another is the health care cost-conscious climate. Managed care insurers, who actively pursue health promotion, ignore the problem of urinary incontinence, do not explain incontinence prevention strategies, and do not embrace effective and proven nonsurgical approaches for incontinence.

To prevent urinary incontinence, public education like the Dry Expectations™ program needs development. Programs addressing normal functioning of the urinary tract and the body's age-related and developmental changes are necessary, as well as information about behavioral changes which details the probability of incontinence. Information concerning access to an appropriate treatment provider is essential for an educated consumer.

Health promotion and prevention strategies for urinary incontinence differ, depending on the specific group at risk. A continence prevention program for a health fitness group includes sessions on pelvic muscle exercises, elimination of caffeine and bladder irritants from the diet, weight management, and adequate fluid intake. On the other hand, a program for women's groups covers changes to the genitourinary tract due to menopause; treatment of urinary tract infections; and constipation and personal hygiene, including preventing perineal skin rashes. Programs for men target prostate disorders and include discussions of the subsequent incontinence that may follow prostate surgery.

Public education is another avenue for health care providers to disseminate information on incontinence. Routine health care visits, health fairs, beauty salons, libraries, and schools provide excellent educational opportunities. School nurses have an opportunity to teach girls about healthy bladder habits, adequate fluid intake, bladder irritants, caffeinated drinks, and pelvic muscle exercises.

An ideal place for promoting bladder health is in senior centers in both urban and rural areas. Persons in centers are vulnerable, as they are at the age when impairments in physical, cognitive, and emotional health develop. The need for continence prevention in this population is immense.

In addition to educating consumers about continence promotion, state governments, employers, industry, and manufacturers must also be educated. The environment where a person works, lives, and socializes has an impact on continence promotion. Adequate toilet facilities that are hygienic, safe, convenient, and private have a direct effect on continence. Work rules, too, affect bladder control. Employment practices that are restrictive and insensitive to employees' basic bladder needs may actually promote incontinence. The arena for health promotion and prevention for the embarrassing and stressful problem of urinary incontinence is expanding. As baby boomers age and become more aware of the problems of incontinence, the demand for programs will increase.

CHAPTER 22

BED-WETTING
AND CHILDREN

Ten percent of all children, mostly boys, over the age of four experience bedtime wetting, or bed-wetting. The problem is usually due to a small bladder. In addition, there are approximately 750,000 children with handicaps and birth defects such as spina bifida who experience ongoing bladder control problems.

CHILDHOOD ENURESIS

Nocturnal enuresis is common in young children. We are all born incontinent. An infant's bladder will empty involuntarily, depending on stimuli and volume. Continence is an adjustment to the social norm. In Western society, the norm for toileting is for women to squat on a commode to void, and men to stand to void. As the toddler's bladder, pelvic nerves, and bladder control center develop, voiding becomes voluntary. Bladder control during the day is usually achieved between the ages of two and three, and at nighttime by age four. However, children may have daytime continence, but lack bladder control during the night. Most children outgrow bed-wetting, but some (around 10 percent) continue during the night. Statistics show that 20 percent of four-year-olds still wet the bed, but that each year 10 to 15 percent of these children stop bed-wetting. Other statistics show that as many as 1 to 3 percent of eighteen-year-olds wet their beds.

Children who wet the bed beyond the age of five generally need more time to have their bladders mature. Nerve pathways between the pelvis and brain may not be fully developed, and these children may have small bladders. Some children sleep so soundly that they don't wake up even when their bladders are full and need to be emptied. A physical problem can also cause bed-wetting, so if it persists past the age of five, you should discuss the situation with your child's pediatrician; bed-wetting can be a symptom of a medical condition such as diabetes or UTI.

Bed-wetting is usually divided into two categories, primary (90 percent) and secondary (5 to 10 percent). Children with primary bed-wetting have never experienced an extended period of dryness (two to three months) without the use of some type of treatment, such as medication. The cause of primary bed-wetting is a bladder that is too small and irritable. Secondary bed-wetting is when the child has been dry for an extended period of time and resumes bed-wetting. Secondary bed-wetting may be caused by diabetes, urinary tract abnormalities, anatomic abnormalities, and psychological factors. In rare cases, bed-wetting can be the result of a narrowing of the end of the urethra. In this situation, stretching of the urethra is done.

Bed-wetting causes social limitations for the child, especially for sleepovers with friends. Parents become frustrated and aggravated over the constant need to change linens. Children and parents have a sense of failure, which can be very painful for the child. As with incontinence in adults, there are myths surrounding bed-wetting in children. Myths include:

MYTH 1: BED-WETTING IN CHILDREN IS NOT A SIGNIFICANT PROBLEM.

Actually it is very significant; 5 to 7 million children in the United States wet their beds, with boys outnumbering girls. Childhood bed-wetting, like adult incontinence, is a hidden problem that few people discuss.

MYTH 2: CHILDREN WHO BED-WET ARE LAZY AND DO IT ON PURPOSE.

Children do not like wet beds! Bed-wetting should not be thought of as a mental, learning, or behavioral problem. The majority of children who bed-wet do not wet by choice to spite their parents, are not lazy, and do not have emotional problems. In general, children are embarrassed by their bed-wetting and feel shame and guilt.

MYTH 3: CHILDREN WHO BED-WET ALL HAVE EMOTIONAL PROBLEMS.

This is not true, as bed-wetting may be caused by hereditary factors. A risk factor for adult incontinence is childhood enuresis. Bed-wetting tends to run in families, and for 70 percent of bed-wetters, you will find that the mother, father, or some other close family member was a bed-wetter as a child.

However, parents need to understand that children will outgrow the problem. Only 5 to 10 percent of children who suffer from enuresis have a physical abnormality. Only 1 percent of adolescents over the age of sixteen are troubled by nocturnal enuresis. There is controversy concerning treatment options; most professionals feel that the parent should wait to take medical action as most children outgrow the problem by puberty.

TREATMENTS

Treatment is directed toward:

- Increasing bladder capacity.
- Increasing awareness of signals from a full bladder.
- Increasing the ability to respond to a bladder contraction by using the outer sphincter muscle to withhold urine (through pelvic exercises).

Diet modification may eliminate bladder irritants, such as foods and drinks that contain caffeine (especially helpful after dinnertime). Some children who have an allergy to milk will improve their bed-wetting problem by eliminating afternoon and evening milk from their diets. Monitor the child's foods and evening snacks for items that may be bladder irritants.

The most often recommended treatment option is behavioral therapy. To increase the amount the bladder can hold, bladder retraining can be taught. This may require charting the number of the child's daytime trips to the bathroom and the time he or she goes to bed. Kegel exercises are also helpful and include teaching the child to interrupt the urinary stream by tightening his or her sphincter muscle. All of these treatments are mentioned in Chapter 14 and can be used in children. If your child wakes up during the night for any reason, teach him or her to always use the toilet. As with all individuals in behavioral training programs, the child must be accountable for his or her behavior. As part of this therapy, it is recommended that the child assume the responsibility of changing the bed linens.

A common approach of behavioral training includes the use of alarm systems, called moisture alarms, that wake the child once wetting begins. Bed-wetting alarms teach the child to wake up before wetting occurs. Alarms and moisture-sensing pads can be purchased through drugstores, medical supply stores, mail-order catalogs, and even through Sears (Lite-Alert® Alarm and Wee-Alert® Alarm) and J.C. Penney (Wet Alarm®). They cost between $45 and $100. These alarms contain a sensor that attaches either to the child's underwear or to the pad on the bed. The alarm will buzz or a sensor will vibrate once the child begins to urinate. You may also try setting an alarm clock to ring every three to four hours, waking the child to urinate. However, many children sleep through the alarm and it only awakens the parent. Many children are scared when they wake up at night and night-lights allow the child to easily see the way to the bathroom. They also remind him to get up and use the toilet.

In children over the age of twelve, drug treatment may be an option. Medications used include:

- Imipramine (Tofranil), is an antidepressant drug which decreases the bladder's irritability and tightens the sphincter. This drug is also used in adults with incontinence. This drug is effective in 75 percent of children; however, once the drug is stopped, the bed-wetting resumes. Another medication that works in a similar fashion is Ditropan.

- DDAVP is a hormone that decreases the amount of urine the body produces at night, thus lessening the chance of bed-wetting. Some research has shown that children who bed-wet may have a deficiency of this hormone, called antidiuretic hormone (ADH). This drug is taken as a nasal spray.

Managing the Wetting

The problem of bed-wetting in a child causes severe disruptions among family members. Most of the parent's frustration is due to the inability to help the child and the daily chore of changing and washing linens. Many times a parent will leave the child in diapers well past the age where they are indicated. It is recommended that you take children out of diapers by the time they are four or five years old and layer the bed with underpads. Many mothers say that Kimberly Clark Pull-Ups® have been a lifesaver, as they provide protection while being acceptable to the child. Never punish your child for wetting the bed; the child cannot control the bed-wetting and punishment usually worsens the problem. In many cases, punishment increases the child's shame and embarrassment. Instead, use positive reinforcement for any success at staying dry. Mark a calendar when the child has a dry night and note the child's success with stars and stickers. This is very effective in decreasing the incidence of bed-wetting. Identifying achievable goals (for example, staying dry one night a week) can be helpful. Try to make it easy for your child to spend the night at a friend's house. Perhaps hiding a Pull-Up® in the bottom of an overnight bag will allow the child to discreetly slip it on. Also, let the friend's parents know about the problem; they are usually very understanding.

FINDING THE PRODUCTS YOU NEED

There are many manufacturers of products, catheters, and devices that can help you manage your problem. All of these products are mentioned in Chapters 16 to 19. These manufacturers have additional educational material on urinary incontinence and their products that they will send you free by calling the numbers indicated. This material will help you understand your incontinence and determine the most appropriate products for management. Most manufacturers are prepared to answer your product-related questions. The following is a list of manufacturers and the products they provide.

3M Health Care
3M Center, Bldg 270-4A-05
St. Paul, MN 55144-1000
(800) 228-3957

3M Health Care has a product line that covers a continuum of care, from healthy skin, to maintenance and prevention for at-risk skin, to early intervention and protection of damaged skin. The skin care program includes the 3M™ No Sting Barrier Film, Antiseptic Skin Cleanser®, Zinc Oxide Vanishing Cream®, Durable Barrier Cream®, A&D Barrier Ointment® and emollient cream.

A+ Medical Products, Inc.
16 Alden Place
West Newton, MA 02165
(888) 843-3334

This company develops medical products that honor women and make a difference in the quality of their lives. Manufactures ASTA-CATH, female catheter guide, the Feminal™ female urinal, and the Belly Bag, a urine collection bag.

Access to Continence Care & Treatment, Inc.
834 Chestnut Street, Suite T172
Philadelphia, PA 19107
(215) 923-1492
website: www.wellweb.com/ACCT/contents.htm

ACCT has available audiocassette tapes that can be used for practicing pelvic muscle exercises. Audiovisual slides and tools are available for professionals for augmenting behavioral training. The Continence Specialist Registry® is a listing of health-care providers who provide services for incontinence.

American Medical Systems, Inc.
10700 Bren Road West
Minnetonka, MN 55343
(800) 328-3881

American Medical Systems is a leading manufacturer of medical devices including artificial urinary sphincters.

Bard Urological Division
Bard Medical Division
Covington, GA 30209
(800) 526-4455

Bard Urological Division is the distributor of Contigen® Bard Collagen Implant, a minimally invasive, nonsurgical outpatient treatment for stress urinary incontinence due to intrinsic sphincter deficiency. Bard manufactureres and distributes the Bard 4-Channel FiberOptic Urodynamic Monitor® as well as a line of pressure sensors and catheters for the diagnostic evaluation of patients with urinary incontinence.

Bard Medical Division supplies a full line of Foley and external catheters, as well as skin care products for incontinence management. Skin care products include Special Care® Cream and Moisture Barrier Ointment, Double Guard® Skin Protectant, Bard Incontinence Protective Barrier Film®, and Medi-Aire® Biological Odor Eliminator.

Caring Products International
200 First Avenue West, Suite 200
Seattle, WA 98119
(800) FEEL DRY (800-333-5397)

Caring Products International distributes Rejoice®, an ultrathin, high-capacity disposable liner with washable cotton pants that look and feel like regular underwear. Rejoice® is currently available to consumers in retail stores.

Coloplast Corporation
1955 West Oak Circle
Marietta, GA 30062-2249
(800) 533-0464

Coloplast Corporation manufactures high-performance urological products under the name Conveen. Conveen has developed Security+ latex-free self-sealing Urisheath external catheters and the Conveen standard urine leg bag with soft fabric backing. The Conveen male external catheters are one- or two-piece systems. Conveen also manufactures intermittent catheters with straight or curved tips. Conveen drip collectors are for men who are experiencing dribbling incontinence.

Coloplast also has a wide variety of skin care products marketed under the name Sween. These products include Baza® Pro Cream, Peri-Wash Skin Care Pack®, Peri-Care®, and Sween Cream®.

ConvaTec
P.O. Box 5254
Princeton, NJ
(800) 422-8811
website: www.convatec.com

ConvaTec, a Bristol-Myers Squibb company, is a leading manufacturer of ostomy, wound, skin, and incontinence care products. The company's products include the ConQuest™ Male Continence System designed for the incontinent active man. The ConQuest™ is a reusable system that uses jockey-style briefs with a pressure pad. The ProSys® Urihesive System NL is a nonlatex hydrocolloid adhesive strip or self-adhering condom catheter system. ConvaTec also has a complete selection of latex external catheters. All ProSys® male external catheters can be attached to the ProSys® leg bag. ConvaTec offers a high quality all silicone Foley catheter that is transparent for the visualization of urine. A Flexi-Seal® fecal collector is available for persons suffering from fecal incontinence. This device is latex free and attached to the skin using adhesives. Vaginal weights called FemTones™ are available as a

safe training aid to help women learn to do pelvic floor exercises properly.
These weights are available in sets of five smooth cones that range in weight
from 20 grams to 70 grams. Each has a cord attached to facilitate removal.
ConvaTec has skin care products under the AloeVesta® name.

Diagnostic Ultrasound, Corp.
18109 NE 76th Street
Redmond, WA 98052
(800) 331-2313

Manufactures the BladderScan™ and BladderManager™ instruments that
measure and monitor bladder volume.

Era III Medical Ltd.
4683 Winterset Drive
Columbus, OH 43220
(800) 838-4823

Distributes a patented treatment protocol called Incon Therapy™ for incontinence. This therapy is a behavioral intervention program that incorpo-
rates EMG biofeedback therapy.

E.K. Johnson
4869 "G" Street
Springfield, OR 97478
(503) 746-6126

E.K. Johnson has a spill-proof rehab urinal for men.

Family Health Media
P.O. Box 1842
Charlottesville, VA 22903
(800) 366-3641

Family Health Media has an excellent video called *Treating Urinary Incontinence,* that was developed for consumers.

Health Services Research & Development, Inc.
10470 Waterfowl Terrace
Columbia, MD 21044
(888) 454-6276

Health Services Research & Development, Inc., developed and markets the Kimbro Comfort Lift (KCL)™ both nationally and internationally since 1986. The inflatable lift can support patients weighing up to 400 pounds. Nurse consultation regarding use of the product is available by phone to customers at no charge.

Hollister, Inc.
InCare Medical Products
2000 Hollister Drive
Libertyville, IL 60048
(800) 323-4060

The Hollister, Inc., product line is a comprehensive offering of systems for the diagnosis, treatment, and continuing care of the incontinent individual. The full line of products includes self-adhesive extended wear external catheters with a non-reflux inner flap, vented urinary leg bags, bedside collectors, female urinary pouches, and fecal incontinence collectors. InCare Medical Products, a division of Hollister, specializes in home- and office-based diagnostic and treatment equipment. The InCare Pelvic Floor Therapy System provides pressure and EMG, biodfeedback, and electrical stimulation therapy for the effective treatment of urinary incontinence.

Humanicare International, Inc.
1471 Jersey Avenue
North Brunswick, NJ 08902
(800) 631-5270

Humanicare has a variety of products which are utilized by many satisfied customers. Products include reusable genderized protective garments, disposable pads, liners, guards, undergarments, diapers, and underpads for adults and children.

INTELLITECS
1 Knollcrest Drive
P.O. Box 371805
Cincinnati, OH 45222-1805
(800) 892-2580

INTELLITECS markets technologically advanced moisture management incontinence products. These products combine the best reusable and disposable innovations to provide great value to the customer, making people's lives more healthy, comfortable, and enjoyable. INTELLITECS has done this by leveraging their excellent heritage and product technology from their parent company, Standard Textile, to create many new and innovative products. Distribution includes pharmacies, Mass Merchants, DME stores, and catalog sales.

Kimberly-Clark Corporation
Consumer Services
P.O. Box 2020
Neenah, WI 54957-2020
(800) 558-6423

Kimberly-Clark Corporation is the manufacturer of Depend® and Poise® absorbent products. For light incontinence Poise® pads are available in several absorbency needs. Depend® Guards for men are designed for light to moderate incontinence. Depend® undergarments for moderate incontinence are available in a button or adjustable strap. Depend® fitted briefs are for regular or overnight absorbency levels and underpads offer protection for bed and other surfaces. Kimberly-Clark is committed to educating consumers and professionals through publication of the *To Life*® magazine, consumer promotions, and the release of a continuing education program, "A Profile of Incontinence," for pharmacists and nurses.

Koregon Enterprises, Inc.
9735 SW Sunshine Court, Suite 100
Beaverton, OR 97005
(800) 544-4240

The Nite Train'r enuresis alarm has a moisture-sensitive pad and alarm that helps the sleeper to wake up during urination.

Mentor Urology
5425 Hollister Avenue
Santa Barbara, CA 93111
(800) 328-3863

Mentor Urology is a leading manufacturer of catheters, primarily intermittent and external. They also distribute skin care products. Their products include the Mentor Self-Cath® which are sterile, latex-free catheters for intermittent and general catheterization. The Female Urine Specimen catheter is one convenient unit for obtaining urine specimens. Mentor has a nice selection of male external catheters that includes the Clear Advantage®, a silicone self-adhering male external catheter; the Freedom Cath®, a self-adhering male external catheter; Uro-San Plus®, a two-piece male external catheter with double-sided adhesive liner and skin shield protective dressing; and Gizmo™, a two-piece, twistproof male external catheter made of pure natural latex. Mentor also has urine collection systems that include the Mentor Male Absorbent Pouch® made from a superabsorbent material that is placed in underwear to collect urine leakage. Mentor's Freedom® leg bag is a soft vinyl bag for use with indwelling catheters. Mentor's skin care products include a three-step skin care kit designed to clean, deodorize, moisturize, and protect affected skin areas.

Milex Products, Inc.
5915 Northwest Highway
Chicago, IL 60631
(800) 621-1278

Distributors of unique gynecologic products including eighteen different type of pessaries, the Kegel perineal exerciser, and exercise Kones.

Nytone Medical Products
2424 South 900 West
Salt Lake City, UT 84119
(801) 973-4090

The Nytone enuretic alarm is a solid-state transistorized enuretic control unit worn on the wrist like a watch. It is completely portable and requires no attachments to the bed. It is absolutely safe for the child. The Nytone alarm is activated by moisture and awakens the sleeper at almost the moment it occurs.

Palco Laboratories
1595 Soquel Drive
Santa Cruz, CA 95065
(800) 346-4488

Palco Laboratories makes the Wet Stop buzzer, which reacts instantly to the first few drops of moisture, teaching a child to stop the flow of urine before the bed becomes wet.

Procter & Gamble Co.
Procter & Gamble Plaza
Cincinnati, OH 45202
(800) 428-8363

Procter & Gamble is another leading manufacturer of consumer incontinence products, Attends®. They provide samples and free information if you write and call.

The Prometheus Group
80 Bow Street
Portsmouth, NH 03801
(800) 442-2325

The Prometheus Group offers the Pathway™ series of EMGs, Synergy™ Plus PC Software, and accessories for the treatment of incontinence that are economical, sophisticated, and user-friendly.

Realmont Ltd.
3300 2nd Street, 12e
Rue St. Hubert
Quebec, Canada J3Y 5K2
(514) 443-2000

Realmont is a Canadian company that makes a female urinal that is specifically for women who are sitting.

Rochester Medical Corporation
1500 2nd Avenue, NW
Stewartville, MN 55976
(800) 243-3315

Rochester Medical offers latex-free, disposable urological and incontinence catheters. Offerings include the Wide Band™ silicone self-adhering male external condom catheter, which features a wide adhesive for greater security. Other male external products offered by Rochester Medical include the Pop-On™, a unique short-sheath silicone catheter, and the Ultraflex® male external catheter that is clear, odorless, and latex-free yet economically priced. In addition to male catheters, Rochester Medical manufactures and markets a full line of clear, 100 percent silicone Foley catheters.

SCA Mölnycke
7030 Louisville Rd.
P.O. Box 90022
Bowling Green, KY 42101
(800) 992-9939

SCA Mölnycke offers a wide selection of innovative products for incontinence and skin care under the PROMISE® brand name. This company was one of the first to introduce a mesh pant with a superabsorbent pad insert.

Sierra Laboratories, Inc.
P.O. Box 27005
Tucson, AZ 85726
(800) 726-2904

Sierra Laboratories, Inc., carries a complete line of urological products for the management of male urinary incontinence. Products include the Comfort Cath SA™, a self-adhering external condom catheter, the Comfort Cath™ a double-sided adhesive strap, and the Comfort Cath™ I, which is a single-sided adhesive strip. Sierra makes Comfort Mate™, a reusable strap that will hold any male external catheter in place without adhesives. The Alpine reusable leg bag, an odor-proof bag, is available through Sierra as are the Uro-Tex® reusable leg bags and the Uro-Tex® McGuire urinal which is washable and reusable. The Manhood™ absorbent pouch can also be obtained through Sierra.

Swiss Medical Products, Inc.
4315 Alpha Road
Dallas, Texas 75244
(800) 633-8872

Swiss Medical Products, Inc., markets a broad line of skin care, wound care, incontinence, and massage products, focusing first on skin care protection. Products include the Elta®seal moisture barrier, Elta®cleanse cleansing foam, Elta® odor eliminator.

TransAqua
P.O. Box 668105
Charlotte, NC 28266-8105
(704) 391-0003

TransAqua's HealthDri® washable incontinence undergarments are individually designed products for men and women with the look and feel of normal underwear. These effective garments, offered in four levels of absorption and three styles, have no pads to add. The HealthDri® moisture management panel captures moisture and moves it away from the skin.

UroMed Corporation
64 A Street
Needham, MA 02194
(888) 987-6633
e-mail: www.uromed.com

UroMed Corporation is the manufacturer of the Reliance® urethral insert and Impress™ miniguard perineal patch. The Reliance® insert is a nonsurgical option for the management of female stress incontinence. Uromed also has an audiovisual program "PelvicFlex" designed to coach woman in learning pelvic muscle exercises. UroMed is the manufacturer of the INTROL™ bladder neck prosthesis which is a new, nonsurgical effective treatment for women with urinary stress incontinence. It reduces UI by providing support to the base of the bladder. It is inserted in the vagina.

UroSurge, Inc.
2660 Crosspark Road
Coralville, Iowa 52241
(800) 658-5965

UroSurge, Inc., is a company developing innovative new products to address the treatment of urinary incontinence. Its first product, the AcuTrainer™, is a beeper-size device for bladder retraining of urge incontinent patients. This device reminds the patient when to void and records voids and any UI episodes. The device provides information to the clinician about compliance, UI episodes, and voiding patterns.

SELF-HELP GROUPS
AND RESOURCES

The following groups can be contacted for more information on urinary incontinence. These groups provide support to women and men with incontinence as well as caregivers.

Agency for Health Care Policy and Research (AHCPR)
Urinary Incontinence Guideline
P.O. Box 8547
Silver Spring, MD 20907
(800) 358-9295
e-mail: AHCPR.gov

The AHCPR was established in 1989 to enhance the quality, appropriateness, and effectiveness of health care in the United States. The AHCPR carries out its mission by conducting and supporting general health services research, including medical effectiveness research, facilitating development of clinical practice guidelines, and disseminating research findings and guidelines to health care providers, policymakers, and the public. The updated urinary incontinence guideline was released in March 1996. (See Appendix C.)

Alliance for Aging
2021 K. Street, NW
Suite 305
Washington, DC 20006
(202) 293-2856

The Alliance for Aging is an organization dedicated to advancing scientific and medical research to improve the health and independence of older Americans.

American Foundation of Urologic Disease
300 W. Pratt Street, Suite 401
Baltimore, Maryland 21201-2463
(800) 242-2383
e-mail: admin@afud.org

The American Foundation for Urologic Disease (AFUD) is dedicated to the prevention and cure of urologic diseases through the expansion of research, education, and public awareness to the general public and health care providers. The Foundation's Health Councils are the nationally recognized clearinghouse for accurate and current information on the following urologic diseases: bladder, prostate, pediatric, kidney, and sexual function. It participates in national awareness campaigns to help patients and their families make more informed treatment decisions.

Continence Restored, Inc.
407 Strawberry Hill Avenue
Stamford, CT 06902
(914) 285-1170

Disseminates information about bladder control to the public and industry and works to establish support groups throughout the United States.

ICIC (IC Information Clearinghouse)
1706 Briery Road
Farmville, VA 23901
(804) 315-0060

Clearinghouse for information on interstitial cystitis (IC)

Interstitial Cystitis Association, Inc. (ICA)
P.O. Box 1553
Madison Square Station
New York, NY 10159
(212) 979-6057
e mail: www.icahelp.com

ICA assists persons with interstitial cystitis (IC) and the medical community in education and research about IC.

National Association for Continence (NAFC)
P.O. Box 8306
Spartansburg, SC 29305-8306
(800) BLADDER (800-252-3337)

The NAFC, formerly Help for Incontinent People (HIP), is a not-for-profit organization dedicated to improving the quality of life of people with incontinence. NAFC's goal is to be the leading source of education, advocacy, and support to the public and to the health professional about the causes, prevention, treatments, and management alternatives for incontinence. In addition to a newsletter and educational brochures, NAFC's services include an audiocassette tape and booklet that coach pelvic muscle exercises, a slide/tape program that health professionals can use in giving talks to patient and community groups, a continence referral service that puts people in touch with local health professionals, and a 100-page resource guide, Products and Services for Incontinence.

National Family Caregivers Association
9621 East Bexhill Drive
Kensington, MD 20895-3104
(800) 896-3650
e-mail: info@nfcacares.org

Dedicated to empower, educate, and support the quality of life of America's 25 million family caregivers.

National Kidney and Urologic Diseases Information Clearinghouse
3 Information Way
Bethesda, MD 20892-3580
(301) 654-4415
e-mail: nkudic@aerie.com

The National Kidney and Urologic Diseases Information Clearinghouse is a service of the National Institute of Diabetes, Digestive, and Kidney Diseases of the National Institutes of Health under the U.S. Public Health Service. Established in 1987, the clearinghouse provides information about diseases of the kidneys and urologic system to the public and professionals. Color pamphlets are available on bladder control in women.

Simon Foundation for Continence
P.O. Box 835
Wilmette, Il 60091
(800) 23-SIMON

The Simon Foundation for Continence is an international not-for-profit organization. Its mission is to bring the problem of incontinence into the open, remove the stigma surrounding it, and provide education for people with incontinence. By calling the toll-free number, you can receive a free information packet that includes a sample of the foundation's newsletter and a list of resource materials. The foundation also coordinates a nationwide network of educational and support groups. This program, called I Will Manage, includes lectures on the causes of and treatments for incontinence. Videos on incontinence and information about bed-wetting are also available.

US-TOO
930 North York Road, Suite 50
Hinsdale, IL 60521-2993
(800) 808-7866

US-TOO is a nonprofit organization that assists prostate cancer survivors in their understanding of the facts and circumstances of their particular situation. US-TOO has 400 chapters throughout the U.S. It holds forums where men and their families can express their feelings and thoughts about prostate disease. It also hosts meetings at which medical professionals speak on various aspects of diagnosis, stages, treatment options, and other related topics. US-TOO's credo is "Learning to Cope Through Knowledge and Hope."

U.S. Department of Health and Human Services
CLINICAL PRACTICE GUIDELINE
"Understanding Incontinence" Patient Booklet

HOW YOUR BODY MAKES, STORES, AND RELEASES URINE

When you eat and drink, your body absorbs the liquid. The kidneys filter out waste products from the body fluids and make urine.

Urine travels down tubes called ureters into a muscular sac called the urinary bladder, which stores the urine.

When you are ready to go to the bathroom, your brain tells your system to relax.

SOURCE: Adapted from U.S. Department of Health and Human Services/Agency for Health Care Policy and Research Publication No. 96-0684, *Clinical Practice Guideline for Acute and Chronic Incontinence* (Consumer Version, Number 2, 1996 update). Used with permission.

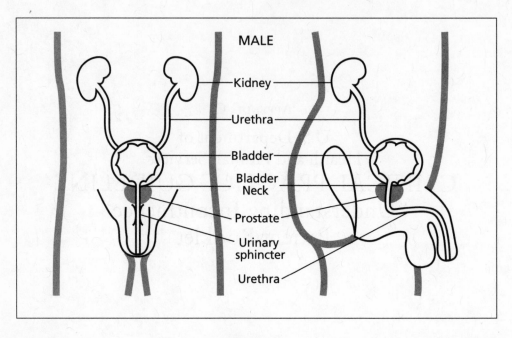

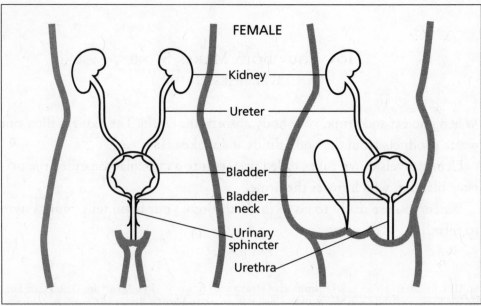

Figure Appendix C.1 The urinary tract

Urine travels out of your bladder through a tube called the urethra. You release urine by relaxing the urethral sphincter and contracting the bladder muscles. The urethral sphincter is a group of muscles that tightens to hold urine in and loosens to let it out.

Understanding Incontinence

Many people lose urine when they don't want to. When this happens enough to be a problem, it is called urinary incontinence.

Urinary incontinence is very common. But some people are too embarrassed to get help. The good news is that millions of men and women are being successfully treated and cured.

Reading this will help you. But it is important to tell your health care provider (such as a doctor or nurse) about the problem. You may even want to bring this booklet with you to help you talk about your incontinence.

Causes of Urinary Incontinence

Urinary incontinence is not a natural part of aging. It can happen at any age, and can be caused by many physical conditions. Many causes of incontinence are temporary and can be managed with simple treatment. Some causes of temporary incontinence are:

- Urinary tract infection
- Vaginal infection or irritation
- Constipation
- Effects of medicine

Incontinence can be caused by other conditions that are not temporary. Other causes of incontinence are:

- Weakness of muscles that hold the bladder in place
- Weakness of the bladder itself
- Weakness of the urethral sphincter muscles
- Overactive bladder muscles
- Blocked urethra (can be from prostate enlargement)
- Hormone imbalance in women
- Neurologic disorders
- Immobility (not being able to move around)

In almost every case, these conditions can be treated. Your health care provider will help to find the exact cause of your incontinence.

Types of Incontinence

There are also many different types of incontinence. Some people have more than one type of incontinence. You should be able to identify the type of incontinence you have by comparing it to the list below.

Urge incontinence: People with urge incontinence lose urine as soon as they feel a strong need to go to the bathroom. If you have urge incontinence you may leak urine:

- When you can't get to the bathroom quickly enough
- When you drink even a small amount of liquid, or when you hear or touch running water

You may also . . .

- Go to the bathroom very often; for example, every two hours during the day and night. You may even wet the bed

Stress incontinence: People with stress incontinence lose urine when they exercise or move in a certain way. If you have stress incontinence, you may leak urine:

- When you sneeze, cough, or laugh
- When you get up from a chair or get out of bed
- When you walk or do other exercise

You may also . . .

- Go to the bathroom often during the day to avoid accidents

Overflow incontinence: People with overflow incontinence may feel that they never completely empty their bladder. If you have overflow incontinence, you may:

- Often lose small amounts of urine during the day and night
- Get up often during the night to go to the bathroom
- Often feel as if you have to empty your bladder but can't
- Pass only a small amount of urine but feel as if your bladder is still partly full
- Spend a long time at the toilet, but produce only a weak, dribbling stream of urine

Some people with overflow incontinence do not have the feeling of fullness, but they lose urine day and night.

Finding the Cause of Urinary Incontinence

Once you tell your health care provider about the problem, finding the cause of your urinary incontinence is the next step.

Your health care provider will talk with you about your medical history and urinary habits. You may be asked to keep a record of your usual habits in a bladder record (see Sample Bladder Record at end of this Appendix). You probably will have a physical examination and urine tests. You may have other tests, as well. These tests will help find the exact cause of your incontinence and the best treatment for you. The table at the end of this booklet lists some of the tests you may be asked to take.

Treating Urinary Incontinence

Once the type and cause of your urinary incontinence are known, treatment can begin. Urinary incontinence is treated in one or more of three ways: behavioral techniques, medication, and surgery.

Behavioral techniques: Behavioral techniques teach you ways to control your own bladder and sphincter muscles (see Figure App. C. 1). They are very simple and work well for certain types of urinary incontinence. Two types of behavioral techniques are commonly used bladder training and pelvic muscle exercises. You may also be asked to change the amount of liquid that you drink. You may be asked to drink more or less water depending on your bladder problem.

Bladder training is used for urge incontinence, and may also be used for stress incontinence. Both men and women can benefit from bladder training. People learn different ways to control the urge to urinate. Distraction (thinking about other things) is just one example. A technique called prompted voiding urinating on a schedule is also used. This technique has been quite successful in controlling incontinence in nursing home patients.

Pelvic muscle exercises called Kegel exercises are used for stress incontinence. The Kegel exercises help to strengthen weak muscles around the bladder.

Medication: Some people need to take medicine to treat conditions that cause urinary incontinence. The most common types of medicine treat infection, replace hormones, stop abnormal bladder muscle contractions, or tighten sphincter muscles. Your health care provider may recommend medication for your condition. You will be taught how and when to take it.

Surgery: Surgery is sometimes needed to help treat the cause of incontinence. Surgery can be used to:

- Return the bladder neck to its proper position in women with stress incontinence
- Remove tissue that is causing a blockage
- Correct severely weakened pelvic muscles
- Enlarge a small bladder to hold more urine

There are many different surgical procedures that may be used to treat incontinence. The type of operation you may need depends on the type and cause of your incontinence. Your doctor will discuss the specific procedure you might need.

Be sure to ask questions so that you fully understand the procedure.

Other Measures and Supportive Devices

Some other products can be used to help manage incontinence. These include pads and catheters. Catheters are used when a person cannot urinate. A catheter is a tube that is placed in the bladder to drain urine into a bag outside the body. The catheter usually is left inside the bladder, but some catheters are not left in. They are put in and taken out of the bladder as needed to empty it every few hours. Condom catheters (mostly used in men) attach to the outside of the body and are not placed directly in the bladder. Specially designed pads are available to help men and women with incontinence.

Catheters and pads are not the first and only treatment for incontinence. They should only be used to make other treatments more effective or when other treatments have failed.

What to Do Next

Your health care provider will tell you about the type of incontinence you have and will recommend a treatment. While you are being treated, be sure to:

- Ask questions
- Follow instructions
- Take all of your medicine
- Report side effects of your medicine, if any
- Report any changes, good and bad, to your health care provider

. . . and remember, incontinence is not a natural part of aging. In most cases, it can be successfully treated and reversed.

Common Tests Used to Diagnose Urinary Incontinence

NAME OF TEST	PURPOSE
Blood tests	Examines blood for levels of various chemicals.
Cystoscopy	Looks for abnormalities in bladder and lower urinary tract. It works by inserting a small tube into the bladder* that has a telescope for the doctor to look through.
Post-void residual (PVR) measurement	Measures how much urine is left in the bladder after urinating Measures how much urine is left in the bladder after urinating by placing a small soft tube into the bladder or by using ultrasound (sound waves).
Stress test	Looks for urine loss when stress is put on bladder muscles usually by coughing, lifting, or exercise.
Urinalysis	Examines urine for signs of infection, blood, or other abnormality.
Urodynamic testing	Examines bladder and urethral sphincter function (may involve inserting a small tube into the bladder; x-rays also can be used to see the bladder).

*Because you may be uncomfortable during this part of the test, you may be given some medication to help relax you.

RISKS AND BENEFITS OF TREATMENT

Three types of treatment are recommended for urinary incontinence:

- Behavioral techniques
- Medicine
- Surgery

How well each of these treatments works depends on the cause of the in-continence and, in some cases, patient effort. The risks and benefits described

SAMPLE BLADDER RECORD

Name: _____ Date: _____

INSTRUCTIONS: Place a check in the appropriate column next to the time you uri-
nated in the toilet or when you had an incontinence episode. Note the reason for
the incontinence and describe your liquid intake (for example, coffee, water) and
estimate the amount (for example, one cup).

Time interval	Urinated in toilet	Had a small episode	Had a large episode	Reason for episode	Type/amount of liquid intake
6–8 A.M.					
8–10 A.M					
4–6 P.M.					
10–noon					
noon–2 P.M.					
2–4 P.M.					
6–8 P.M.					
8–10 P.M.					
10–midnight					
overnight					

No. of pads used today: _____ No. of episodes: _____

Comments: _____
_____
_____
_____
_____

Adapted from: U.S. Department of Health and Human Services/Agency for Health Care Policy
and Ressearch Publication No. 96-0684, Clinical Practice Guideline for Acute and Chronic Incontinence (Consumer Version, Number 2, 1996 update).

below are based on current medical knowledge and expert opinion. How well a treatment works may also depend on the individual patient. A treatment that works for one patient may not be as effective for another patient. Therefore, it is important to talk with a health care provider about treatment choices.

Behavioral techniques. There are no risks for this type of treatment.

Medicine. As with most drugs, there is a risk of having a side effect. If you are taking medicine for other conditions, the drugs could react with each other. Therefore, it is important to work with the health care provider and report all of your medicines and any side effects as soon as they happen.

Surgery. With any surgery there is a possibility of a risk or complication. It is important to discuss these risks with your surgeon.

PELVIC MUSCLE (KEGEL) EXERCISES
Patient Teaching Tool

How to Find the Pelvic Muscle

Imagine you are at a party and the rich food you have just eaten causes you to have gas. The muscle that you use to hold back gas is the pelvic muscle. Some people find this muscle by trying to stop their stream of urine. Another way to find the muscle is by pulling your rectum, vagina, or urethra up inside your body.

Exercising the Muscle

Begin by emptying your bladder. Then try to relax completely. Tighten your pelvic muscle and hold for a count of 10 or for 10 seconds, then relax the muscle completely for a count of 10 or for 10 seconds. You should feel a lifting sensation in the area around the vagina or a pulling in your rectum.

What if I Cannot Squeeze for 10 Seconds?

At first you may not be able to squeeze for a count of 10, so squeeze for a count of 5 and relax for 5. In time increase squeezing to 10 seconds. If the muscle starts to tire after six or eight exercises, stop and go back to exercising later.

When to Exercise

Do these exercise three times a day, 10 exercises in the morning, 10 in the afternoon, and 15 at night. Or you can exercise for 10 minutes, three times a day. You can use a kitchen timer to time yourself.

Common Mistakes

Never use your stomach, legs, or buttocks muscles. Put your hand on your stomach when you squeeze your pelvic muscle. If you feel your stomach move, then you are also using these muscles. Your legs and buttocks muscles should not move.

Where to Practice These Exercises

These exercises can be practiced anywhere and anytime. Most people like to exercise while lying on their bed or sitting in a chair. Women can even do these exercises during sexual intercourse. Tighten pelvic muscles to grip your partner's penis and then relax. Your partner should be able to feel an increase in pressure. If you have a "bladder exercise" tape, listen to it twice a day and follow the instructions.

Can These Exercises Hurt Me?

No! These exercises cannot hurt you in any way. Most patients find them relaxing and easy. If you get back pain or stomach pain after you exercise, then you are probably trying too hard and using stomach muscles. If you experience headaches then you are also tensing your chest muscles and probably holding your breath.

When Will I Notice a Change?

After four to six weeks of consistent daily exercise, you will begin to notice less urinary leakage, and after three months you will see an even bigger difference. Make these exercises part of your lifestyle, tighten the muscle when you walk, before you cough, as you stand up, and on the way to the bathroom.

GLOSSARY

ABSORBENT PRODUCTS: Pads and garments, either disposable or reusable, worn to contain urinary incontinence or uncontrolled urine leakage. Absorbent products include shields, guards, undergarment pads, combination pad-panty systems, diaperlike garments, and bed pads.

ACETYLCHOLINE: A substance that plays an important part in the transmission of nerve impulses in the parasympathetic nervous system. This system controls smooth muscles, including those of the bladder and urethra.

ACUTE INCONTINENCE: Incontinence that comes on suddenly, usually caused by a new illness or condition and often easily reversed with appropriate treatment of the condition that caused it.

ANAL SPHINCTERS: The muscles in the anus.

ANTICHOLINERGIC: A drug that interferes with the effects of acetylcholine.

ANTI-INCONTINENCE SURGERY: The use of surgical procedures to treat urinary incontinence (*see* artificial urinary sphincter, bladder suspension, periurethral bulking injections, sling procedures).

ANUS: The final 2 inches of the rectum, surrounded by the internal anal sphincter and the external sphincter.

Artificial urinary sphincter: A mechanical device surgically implanted into the patient that consists of a cuff, placed around the bulbar urethra or bladder neck, a pressure-regulating balloon, and a pump. The device is used to control opening and closing of the urethra manually and is the most commonly used surgical procedure for the treatment of male urethral insufficiency.

Atonic bladder: Also referred to as a lower motor neuron bladder. Often caused by peripheral neuropathies, such as diabetes mellitus. The bladder is flaccid and overdistended with urine. Overflow incontinence may occur.

Autoimmune: A condition in which the body produces antibodies to its own tissue.

Bacteria: Microscopic organisms that can cause infection and are usually treated with antibiotics.

Bedside commode: A portable toilet used by individuals who have difficulty ambulating to standard facilities.

Behavioral techniques: Specific interventions designed to alter the relationship between the patient's symptoms and his/her behavior and/or environment for the treatment of maladaptive urinary voiding patterns. This may be achieved by modification of the behavior and/or environment of the patient (*see* biofeedback, bladder training, electrical stimulation, habit training, pelvic muscle exercises, prompted voiding).

Benign prostatic hyperplasia (BPH): A common disorder of men over the age of fifty characterized by enlargement of the prostate, which may press against the urethra and interfere with the flow of urine and cause overflow incontinence. BPH is the most common cause of such anatomic obstruction in elderly men.

Biofeedback therapy: A behavioral technique in which a person learns how to consciously control involuntary responses such as muscle contractions. The person receives a visual, auditory, or tactile signal (the feedback) that indicates how well the person's muscles are responding to the commands of the persons's nervous system. The signal is derived from a measurable physiologic parameter, which is subsequently used in an educational process to accomplish a specific therapeutic result. The signal is displayed in a quantitative way, and the patient is taught how to alter it and thus control the physiologic process.

BLADDER: The bladder is a muscular organ which lies in the pelvis and is supported by the pelvic floor muscles. The bladder has only two functions; to stretch to allow the storage of urine and to contract to enable the expulsion of urine. The term detrusor is used to refer to the smooth muscle structure of the bladder.

BLADDER CATHETER: A narrow flexible tube inserted into the urethra and into the bladder for the purpose of draining urine or performing diagnostic tests of bladder or urethral function.

BLADDER CATHETERIZATION: A procedure in which a catheter is passed through the urethra and into the bladder for the purpose of draining urine and performing diagnostic tests of bladder or urethral function.

BLADDER DIARY OR RECORD: A daily record of bladder habits, documenting urination and episodes of incontinence.

BLADDER SUSPENSION: Also called bladder neck suspension. A term for several surgical procedures employed to treat urethral hypermobility by elevating and securing the bladder to its proper position within the body. The two major types of bladder suspension surgical procedures are:

Retropubic suspension: Consists of several different surgical techniques performed through a low abdominal incision. All techniques are designed to elevate the lower urinary tract within the retropubic space, differing only in the structures used to achieve the elevation.

Needle bladder neck suspension: Consists of several different surgical techniques performed through a vaginal approach and small low abdominal incision; all involve the use of a long needle to transfer the sutures adjacent to the urethra and bladder neck through the retropubic space into the abdominal wall anterior to the rectus fascia, where the sutures are fastened or anchored.

BLADDER TRAINING: A behavioral technique that requires the patient to resist or inhibit the sensation of urgency (the strong desire to urinate), to postpone voiding, and to urinate according to a timetable rather than the urge to void.

BOWEL MOVEMENT: The act of passing feces through the anus.

BOWELS: Another word for intestines.

CANCER: Uncontrolled proliferation of abnormal cells that if left untreated takes control of an entire organ or even the entire body.

CATHETERIZATION: Techniques for managing urinary incontinence that involve the use of a slender tube inserted through the urethra or through the anterior abdominal wall into the bladder, urinary reservoir, or urinary conduit to allow urine drainage (*see* indwelling catheters, intermittent catheterization).

CHOLINERGIC: Fibers in the parasympathetic nervous system that release acetylcholine.

CLINICAL PRACTICE GUIDELINES: A set of systematically developed statements or recommendations designed to assist practitioner and patient decisions about appropriate health care for specific clinical circumstances. Such guidelines are designed to assist health care practitioners in the prevention, diagnosis, treatment, and management of specific clinical conditions.

COMPRESSION DEVICE (PENILE CLAMP): A device used to put direct pressure on the outside of the urethra causing it to remain closed until the device is removed and the bladder is allowed to drain.

CONDOM CATHETERS: A condomlike device placed over the penis to allow bladder drainage and collection of urine (*see* external condom catheters).

CONSTIPATION: A condition in which bowel movements are infrequent, hard, and dry, and elimination of feces is difficult.

CONTINENCE: The ability to exercise voluntary control over the urge to urinate or defecate until an appropriate time and place can be found to do so.

CYSTITIS: Irritation or inflammation (swelling) of the bladder, usually caused by an infection.

CYSTOCELE: An intrusion or bulging of the bladder into the vagina, usually caused when the vaginal muscles that support the bladder and urethra are stretched or damaged. Urine can pool or collect in the sac that protrudes, becoming stagnant and serving as a convenient place for bacteria to grow. Women with a cystocele may have repeated bladder infections.

CYSTOMETRY: A test used to assess the function of the bladder by measuring the pressure/volume as the bladder is slowly being filled. Cystometry is used to assess detrusor activity, sensation, capacity, and compliance. There are different variations of the test depending on the problem being investigated, but all involve insertion of a catheter into the bladder.

CYSTOURETHROGRAPHY: The use of X-ray imaging to examine the urinary bladder and urethra. In voiding cystourethrography, an X-ray picture of the bladder and urethra is obtained during urination.

CYSTOSCOPY: Also called cystourethroscopy. A procedure used to diagnose urinary tract disorders and provide a direct view of the urethra and bladder by inserting a flexible scope into the urethra and then into the bladder.

DECREASED BLADDER COMPLIANCE: A failure to store urine in the bladder caused by the loss of bladder wall elasticity and of bladder accommodation. This condition may result from radiation cystitis or from inflammatory bladder conditions such as chemical cystitis, interstitial cystitis, and certain neurologic bladder disorders.

DEFECATE: The act of having a bowel movement.

DEHYDRATION: A state that occurs when insufficient fluid is present to fulfill the body's fluid needs.

DEMENTIA: General loss of short- and long-term memory and mental deterioration. It may affect emotions, abstract thinking, judgment, impulse control, and learning and can cause functional incontinence.

DETRUSOR: In the urinary system, the detrusor muscle is the smooth muscle in the wall of the bladder that contracts the bladder and expels the urine.

DETRUSOR SPHINCTER DYSSYNERGIA (DSD): An inappropriate contraction of the external sphincter concurrent with an involuntary contraction of the detrusor. In the adult, DSD is a common feature of neurologic voiding disorders.

DETRUSOR HYPERACTIVITY WITH IMPAIRED BLADDER CONTRACTILITY (DHIC): A condition characterized by involuntary detrusor contractions in which patients either are unable to empty their bladders completely or can empty their bladders completely only with straining, due to poor contractility of the detrusor.

DETRUSOR INSTABILITY (UNSTABLE BLADDER): Involuntary detrusor contraction in the absence of associated neurologic disorders (*see* urge incontinence).

DIABETIC NEUROPATHY: A condition in which portions of the spinal cord and its nerves have degenerated as a result of diabetes.

DISIMPACTION: The act of removing stool from the rectum which has not been eliminated normally. Enemas, suppositories, laxatives, and finger extraction are all means of disimpacting stool.

DIURETIC: An agent that increases urination.

DYSURIA: Painful or difficult urination, most frequently caused by infection or inflammation; can also be caused by certain drugs.

ELECTRICAL STIMULATION: The application of electric current to stimulate or inhibit the pelvic floor muscles or their nerve supply in order to induce a direct therapeutic response.

ELECTROLYTES: An element or compound that when melted or dissolved in water breaks up into atoms that are able to carry an electric charge. Electrolyte amounts vary in a person's blood. Examples of eletrolytes are calcium, potassium, and sodium.

ELECTROMYOGRAPHY (EMG): A diagnostic test that is used to measure the electrical activity of the muscles.

ENURESIS: Involuntary loss of urine (urinary incontinence) during sleep. This term is most often applied to bed-wetting in children, or nocturnal enuresis.

ESTROGEN: A hormone produced primarily by the ovaries. Estrogen is believed to play a major role in maintaining the strength and tone of the pelvic floor.

EVACUATION: Another word for bowel movement.

External condom catheters: Devices for externally draining the bladder made from latex rubber, polyvinyl, or silicone that are secured on the shaft of the penis by some form of adhesive and are connected to urine collecting bags by a tube.

EXTERNAL SPHINCTER: Band of muscle downstream from the internal sphincter responsible for maintaining urinary incontinence.

FASCIA: Tissue of the body that connects to structures such as bone, tendons, and ligaments.

FECAL IMPACTION: A mass of stool that remains packed in the rectum rather than being passed normally. Impaction can contribute to incontinence by irritating the urethra, causing urge UI, or by blocking the urethra and preventing the bladder from emptying completely, causing overflow incontinence.

Fecal incontinence: The accidental and involuntary loss of liquid or solid stool or gas from the anus.

Feces: Waste material from the intestines. Feces are composed of bacteria, undigested food, and material sloughed from the intestines.

Flatulence: The release of gas through the anus.

Gas: Material that results from swallowed air or that is created when bacteria in the colon break down waste material. Gas that is released from the rectum is called flatulence.

Habit training: A behavioral technique that calls for scheduled toileting at regular intervals on a planned basis to prevent incontinence. Unlike bladder training, there is no systematic effort to motivate the patient to delay voiding and resist the urge.

Hematuria: Blood in the urine.

Hesitancy: Difficulty starting the urine stream, or increase in length of time between initiation of urination by relaxation of the urethral sphincter and when urine stream actually begins.

Hydronephrosis: Dilation of the renal pelvis and calices and, sometimes, collecting ducts, secondary to obstruction of urine flow by calculi, tumors, neurologic disorders, or various congenital anomalies.

Hyperreflexia: Any exaggeration of reflexes. In urinary incontinence, an involuntary detrusor contraction resulting from a neurologic disorder.

Impaction: A blockage in the rectum composed of a large amount of dried stool that is difficult to evacuate.

Incontinence: The accidental or involuntary loss of urine or stool. A person may have urinary or fecal incontinence or both (sometimes called double incontinence).

INDWELLING CATHETERS: Tube devices inserted into the bladder to drain the urine continuously.

INTERMITTENCY: Interruption of urinary stream while voiding.

INTERMITTENT CATHETERIZATION: The use of catheters inserted through the urethra into the bladder every three to six hours for bladder drainage in persons with urinary retention.

INTRINSIC SPHINCTER DEFICIENCY (ISD): A cause of stress urinary incontinence in which the urethral sphincter is unable to contract and generate sufficient resistance in the bladder, especially during stress maneuvers. ISD may be due to congenital sphincter weakness, such as myelomeningocele or epispadias, or it may be acquired subsequent to prostatectomy, trauma, radiation therapy, or sacral cord lesions.

INVOLUNTARY DETRUSOR CONTRACTION: A cause of urinary incontinence resulting from uncontrolled contractions of the detrusor.

KIDNEY: One of two paired organs that continually filter the blood to separate out waste products, which are combined with excess water to form urine.

MEATUS: The opening to the urethra.

MICTURITION: Another term for urination or voiding.

MINIMUM DATA SET (MDS): A federally mandated screening and assessment form for Medicare- and Medicaid-certified long-term care facilities in the United States. This form is completed within fourteen days of admission to the facility, quarterly, and when there is a significant change in the resident's status. An annual update is also required. The information collected in the MDS is used in planning the individual's care.

MIXED URINARY INCONTINENCE: The combination in a patient of urge urinary incontinence and stress urinary incontinence (*see* urge incontinence, stress incontinence).

NERVOUS SYSTEM: The voluntary and involuntary nervous systems are composed of the brain, the spinal cord, and the sensory nerves, which provide messages to the brain from the body, and motor nerves, which provide messages from the brain to the muscles and which help muscles function.

NEUROGENIC BLADDER: An atonic or unstable bladder associated with a neurological condition, such as diabetes, stroke, or spinal cord injury.

NOCTURIA: Being awakened at night by the urge to urinate.

OVERACTIVE BLADDER: A condition characterized by involuntary detrusor contractions during the bladder filling phase, which may be spontaneous or provoked and which the patient cannot suppress.

OVERFLOW INCONTINENCE: The involuntary loss of urine associated with overdistension of the bladder. Overflow incontinence results from urinary retention that causes the capacity of the bladder to be overwhelmed. Continuous or intermittent leakage of a small amount of urine results.

PELVIC FLOOR: A muscular structure that plays an important role in maintaining continence in males and female. It forms a hammock slung from the front of the pelvis to the back. It supports the organs of the pelvis——the bladder, uterus, and rectum.

PELVIC FLOOR MUSCLES: The hammock or sling of muscles in the pelvic floor that normally assist in maintaining continence by supporting the pelvic organs.

PELVIC MUSCLE EXERCISES (PMEs): A behavioral technique that requires repetitive active exercise of the pubococcygeus muscle to improve urethral resistance and urinary control by strengthening the periurethral and pelvic muscles. Also called Kegel exercises or pelvic floor exercises.

PELVIS: The ring of bones at the lower end of the trunk in which the pelvic organs lie.

PERINEOMETER: An instrument originally invented by Dr. Arnold Kegel to measure the strength of pelvic muscle contractions. An electronic perineometer is used in EMG biofeedback training.

PERINEUM: Area between the anus and vagina in women, and anus and base of penis in men.

PERIURETHRAL BULKING INJECTIONS: A surgical treatment for urethral sphincter insufficiency that involves injecting materials such as polytetrafluoroethylene (PTFE) or collagen into the periurethral area to increase urethral compression.

PESSARIES: Devices for women that are placed intravaginally to treat pelvic relaxation or prolapse of pelvic organs.

PHARMACOLOGIC TREATMENT: The use of medications to treat urinary incontinence.

POLYURIA: Excretion of a large volume of urine during a certain interval of time. It can be a result of uncontrolled diabetes mellitus or the administration or a diuretic.

POSTVOID RESIDUAL (PVR) VOLUME: The amount of fluid remaining in the bladder immediately following the completion of urination. Estimation of PVR volume can be made by abdominal palpation and percussion or bimanual examination. Specific measurement of PVR volume can be accomplished by catheterization, pelvic ultrasound, radiography, or radioisotope studies.

PREVALENCE: Number of cases of a disease existing in a population at a given time.

PROLAPSE: The protrusion of the uterus, rectum, or bladder into the vagina.

PROMPTED VOIDING: A behavioral technique for use primarily with dependent or cognitively impaired persons. Prompted voiding attempts to teach the incontinent person awareness of his/her incontinence status and to request toileting assistance, either independently or after being prompted by a caregiver.

PROSTATE: A donut-shaped gland found only in men that surrounds the urethra between the bladder and the pelvic floor.

PROSTATITIS: Irritation or inflammation of the prostate.

PUBOCOCCYGEUS MUSCLE: Another name for the levator ani muscle, one of the pelvic muscles that hold the pelvic organs in place.

PUDENDAL NERVE: Main nerve supplying the pelvic floor, bladder, and urethra. Damage to this nerve can cause incontinence.

RECTOCELE: Bulging of the rectum into the space normally occupied by the vagina, suggesting weakness of the pelvic floor.

RECTUM: Last segment of colon, or large intestine; the lowest part of the bowel found right before the anus.

RESIDENT ASSESSMENT PROFILE (RAP): Part of the minimum data set that assists the nurse to assess the cause of various disruptions or conditions. The RAP provides a systematic method of assessment and is used in the development of an individual's care plan.

RETENTION: Inability to empty urine from the bladder, which can be caused by atonic bladder or obstruction of the urethra.

RISK FACTOR: Quality that makes a person more susceptible to a specific disease.

SCHEDULED TOILETING: Assistance to toilet or use of bedpan or urinal offered on a fixed schedule; for example, every two to four hours.

SENSORY URGENCY: Urgency associated with bladder hypersensitivity (*see* urge/urgency).

SLING PROCEDURES: Surgical methods for treating urinary incontinence involving the placement of a sling, made either of tissue obtained from the patient or from another source, under the urethrovesical junction and anchored to retropubic and/or abdominal structures.

STRESS URINARY INCONTINENCE: A form of urinary incontinence characterized by the involuntary loss of urine from the urethra during physical exertion; for example, during coughing. The stress incontinence symptom or complaint may be confirmed by observing urine loss coincident with an increase in abdominal pressure in the absence of a detrusor contraction or an overdistended bladder (*see* hypermobility of bladder neck, intrinsic sphincter deficiency).

STRESS MANEUVERS: Activities that increase pressure in the bladder, such as coughing and laughing; this is a diagnostic test to check for stress UI.

SUPRAPUBIC: Above the pubic bone.

SUPRAPUBIC CYSTOSTOMY: A surgical procedure involving insertion of a tube or similar instrument through the anterior abdominal wall above the symphysis pubis into the bladder to permit urine drainage from the bladder.

TRANSIENT URINARY INCONTINENCE: Temporary episodes of urinary incontinence that are reversible once the cause or causes of the episode(s) are identified and treated.

TRIGONE: The most sensitive area on the inside (wall) of the bladder, where bladder nerves are highly concentrated.

ULTRASONOGRAPHY: A technique that uses ultrasound to obtain visual images of the urinary tract for the purpose of assessing its anatomic status.

UNDERACTIVE BLADDER: A condition characterized by a bladder contraction of inadequate magnitude and/or duration to effect bladder emptying in a normal time span. This condition can be caused by drugs, fecal impaction, and neurologic conditions such as diabetic neuropathy or low spinal cord injury, or as a result of radical pelvic surgery. It also can result from a weakening of the detrusor muscle from vitamin B_{12} deficiency or idiopathic causes.

Bladder underactivity may cause overdistension of the bladder, resulting in overflow incontinence (*see* overflow incontinence).

Ureters: Two very thin muscular tubes about 8 or 9 inches long that transport urine from the kidneys to the bladder.

Urethra: A narrow tube through which urine flows from the bladder to the outside of the body; the opening of the urethra is at the end of the penis in men and just above the vaginal opening in women.

Urethral dilatation: A procedure in which a metal rod, called a dilator, is passed through the urethra for the purpose of opening a urethral stricture.

Urethral obstruction: Blockage of the urethra causing difficulty with urination; usually caused by a stricture or in men by an enlarged prostate.

Urethral stricture: Narrowing of the urethra.

Urethral pressure profilometry (UPP): A technique used to measure resting and dynamic pressures in the urethra.

Urethral sphincter mechanism: The segment of the urethra that influences storage and emptying of urine in the bladder. It controls bladder voiding by relaxing, which opens the outlet from the bladder, allowing urine to flow from the bladder to the outside of the body. A deficiency of the urethral sphincter mechanism may allow leakage of urine in the absence of a detrusor contraction.

Urethrocele: A hernia in which part of the urethra presses on the vaginal wall.

Urge: The sensation from the bladder producing the desire to void.

Urge incontinence: The involuntary and accidental loss of urine when the person is aware of the need to get to the bathroom but is not able to hold the urine long enough to get there. Usually it is associated with an abrupt and strong desire to void (urgency). Urge incontinence is usually correlated with urodynamic findings of involuntary detrusor contractions or detrusor over-activity (*see* detrusor external sphincter dyssynergia, detrusor hyperactivity with impaired bladder contractility, detrusor instability, hyperreflexia, sensory urgency).

URGENCY: A strong, intense, and often sudden desire to void.

URINARY INCONTINENCE (UI): Involuntary or accidental loss of urine sufficient to be a problem. There are several types of UI, but all are characterized by an inability to restrain or control urinary voiding (*see* mixed urinary incontinence, nocturnal enuresis, overflow incontinence, stress incontinence, transient urinary incontinence, urge incontinence).

URINARY TRACT: Passageway from the kidney to the urinary orifice through the ureters, bladder, and urethra.

URINARY TRACT INFECTION (UTI): An infection in the urinary tract caused by the invasion of disease-causing microorganisms, which proceed to establish themselves, multiply, and produce various symptoms in their host. Infection of the bladder, better known as cystitis, is particularly common in women, mainly because of the much shorter urethra, which provides less of a barrier to bacteria. In men, infection is usually associated with obstruction to the flow of urine, such as prostate gland enlargement.

URINATE: To void or to pass urine.

URINATION: The act of passing urine.

URINE: Waste products filtered from the blood and combined with excess water by the kidneys.

URODYNAMIC TESTS: Tests designed to duplicate as nearly as possible the symptoms of incontinence in the way that the patient actually experiences them. These tests determine the anatomic and functional status of the urinary bladder and urethra (*see* cystometry, electromyography, urethral pressure profilometry, uroflowmetry, videourodynamics).

Uroflowmetry: A urodynamic test that measures urine flow either visually, electronically, or with the use of a disposable flowmeter unit.

Uterine prolapse: The uterus has slipped (dropped) from its normal position and the cervix is closer to or may protrude outside the vagina.

Vagina: Also known as the birth canal. The vagina is a collapsible tube of smooth muscle with its opening located between the urethral orifice and the anal sphincter of women.

Valsalva maneuver: The action of closing the airways and straining down on the abdominal muscles (such as when straining to have a bowel movement).

Videourodynamics: A technique that combines the various urodynamic tests with simultaneous fluoroscopy. Fluoroscopy is a technique for examining internal structures by viewing the shadows cast on a fluorescent screen by objects or parts through which X-rays are directed.

Voiding or bladder diary (record): Also called an incontinence chart. A record maintained by the patient or caregiver that is used to record the frequency, timing, amount of voiding, and/or other factors associated with the patient's urinary incontinence.

Voiding reflex: The reflex in which the bladder indicates to the spinal cord that it is full of urine and the spinal cord then signals the bladder to contract and empty.

SELECTED READINGS

AGENCY FOR HEALTH CARE POLICY AND RESEARCH. "Alert for Directors of Nursing: Establishing, Implementing and Continuing an Effective Continence Program in a Long-Term Care Facility." Rockville, Md.: United States Department of Health and Human Services. Public Health Service, AHCPR Publication No. 96-0063. August, 1996.

———. "Helping People with Incontinence," *Clinical Practice Guideline, Caregiver Guide*, No 2, 1996 Update, Rockville, Md.: United States Department of Health and Human Services. Public Health Service, AHCPR Publication No. 96-0683. August 1996.

———. "Managing Acute and Chronic Urinary Incontinence," *Clinical Practice Guideline, Quick Reference Guide for Clinicians*, No 2, 1996 Update, Rockville, Md.: United States Department of Health and Human Services. Public Health Service, AHCPR Publication No. 96-0686. March 1996.

———. "Understanding Incontinence," *Clinical Practice Guideline, Patient Guide*, No 2, 1996 Update, Rockville, Md.: United States Department of Health and Human Services. Public Health Service, AHCPR Publication No. 96-0684. March 1996.

———. "Urinary Incontinence in Adults: Acute and Chronic Management," *Clinical Practice Guideline*, No 2, 1996 Update, Rockville, Md.: United States

DEPARTMENT OF HEALTH AND HUMAN SERVICES. Public Health Service, AHCPR Publication No. 96-0682. March 1996.

BRUNING, NANCY, *What You Can Do About Bladder Control*. New York: Dell Publishing, 1992.

BURGER, S.G., V. FRASER, S. HUNT, AND B. FRANK. *Nursing Homes, Getting Good Care There*. American Source Books, Impact Publishers, 1996.

BURGIO K.L., K.L. PEARCE, AND A.J. LUCCO. *Staying Dry, A Practical Guide to Bladder Control*. Baltimore: Johns Hopkins University Press, 1989.

CHALKER, R., AND K. WHITMORE. *Overcoming Bladder Disorders*. New York: Harper Perennial, 1990.

EICHENBAUM, K. *The Toilets of New York*. Wisconsin: Litterati Books, 1990.

KORDA, M. *Man to Man: Surviving Prostate Cancer*. New York: Random House, 1996.

LUSTBADER, W., AND N.R. HOOYMAN. *Taking Care of Aging Family Members*. New York: The Free Press, 1994.

NATIONAL KIDNEY AND UROLOGIC DISEASES ADVISORY BOARD. "Barriers to Rehabilitation of Persons with End-Stage Renal Disease or Chronic Urinary Incontinence." Workshop summary report. March 7–9, 1994. Bethesda, Maryland.

ROB, C. *The Caregivers Guide*. Boston: Houghton Mifflin, 1991.

SCHUSTER, M.M., AND J. WEHMUELLER. *Keeping Control: Understanding and Overcoming Fecal Incontinence*. Baltimore: Johns Hopkins University Press, 1994.

INDEX

for women, 224-225

Dexterity, manual, 121

Diabetes, 74

Diapers, 39

Diarrhea, 97-100

    prolonged, 100

    treatment, 100

Diary, bladder, 125-131

Diet, 80-81, 143-146

Disabilities, physical, 49, 56

Diseases

    Alzheimer's, 72-73

    chronic, 42

    Parkinson's, 75-76

    and related causes, 71-86

Disposal, trash, 2

Ditropan, 176

Diuretics, 43, 53-54

DMEs (medical equipment dealers), 189

Doctors, 106, 108-110

    family doctors, 109

    geriatricians, 109

    gynecologists, 109-110

    urologists, 110

Double voiding, 78

Drainage bags, caring, 209-213

Drainage tube, 10

Drugs; *See also* Hormones; Medications

    bethanechol, 177

    Ditropan, 176

    flavoxate, 176

    hycosamine, 176

    hyoscyamine sulfate, 176

    imipramine, 176, 293

    oxybutinin, 176

    Pro-Banthine, 177

    propantheline, 177

    sympathomimetic, 177

    Tofranil, 176, 293

    Urispas, 176

Dry Expectations, 284-286

E

Edema, 121

EMG (electromyographic) probe, 165

Enemas, 96

Enuresis, childhood, 289-292

Environmental barriers, 44, 55-57

Episiotomy, 46

Estrogen, 14, 46, 122, 178-179

ET (enterostomal therapy) nurses, 111

Europe, 30

Examination, 121-123

    genital, 123

    pelvic, 122-123

    rectal, 123

    stomach, 121

Excursions, 29-30

Exercises, 22, 94, 157-162

F

Family doctors, 109

Family members, helping, 265-267

Fecal impaction, 101-102

Feedback, positive, 281

Female hormones, 178-179

Fiber-rich foods, 92-93